NANDA

NURSING DIAGNOSES:
DEFINITIONS &
CLASSIFICATION

2001–2002

W9-CYS-742

NANDA

NURSING DIAGNOSES:

DEFINITIONS & CLASSIFICATION

2001–2002

North American Nursing Diagnosis Association
Philadelphia

For information, contact NANDA, 1211 Locust Street, Philadelphia PA 19107, USA
Telephone: 215.545.7222/800.647.9002.
Fax: 214.545-8107. E-mail: NANDA@rmpinc.com.
Web site: www.NANDA.org

Printed in the United States of America
10 9 8 7 6 5 4 3 2 1

ISBN 0.9637042.7.3

Contents

Preface, vii
Introduction, ix
  How to Use This Book, x

Part 1 NANDA Nursing Diagnoses, 2001–2002   **1**
  Table 1.1 Nomenclature Conversion: Taxonomy I
    to Taxonomy II, 3
  NANDA Nursing Diagnoses With Definitions,
    Defining Characteristics or Risk Factors, and
    Related Factors, 13

Part 2 Taxonomy II   **209**
  History of the Development of Taxonomy II, 211
  Structure of Taxonomy II, 212
  Definitions of the Axes, 213
  Figure 2.1 Taxonony II: Domains and Classes, 214
  Table 2.1 Taxonomy I: Domains, Classes,
    Diagnostic Concepts, and Diagnoses, 221
  Further Development of Taxonomy II Nursing
    Diagnoses, 232
  Code Conversion: Taxonomy I to Taxonomy II, 232
  Table 2.2 Code Conversion: Taxonomy I to
    Taxonomy II, 233

Part 3 Nursing Diagnosis Development   **239**
  Diagnosis Submission Guidelines, 241
  Diagnosis Staging Criteria, 242
  Glossary of Terms Used by NANDA, 245

  NANDA Guidelines for Copyright Permission, 247
  NANDA Board of Directors, 248
  NANDA Diagnosis Review Committee, 248
  NANDA Taxonomy Committee, 248
  Nursing Diagnosis Extension and Classification (NDEC)
    Research Team, 248
  An Invitation to Join NANDA, 250
  NANDA Membership Application, 252
  Index, 253

Preface

Making a nursing diagnosis requires analysis, synthesis, and accuracy in interpreting and making sense of complex clinical data. This critical thinking process allows the nurse to make decisions about desired outcomes and interventions needed to help achieve those outcomes. However, unless the nurse can document his or her thinking in a manner other nurses and healthcare providers can interpret, that thinking process is invisible. Accurately naming and reporting the results of the nurse's critical thinking helps other caregivers know a patient's needs and how the plan of care will help meet those needs. Using standardized nursing language to document the nurse's thinking is an efficient way to achieve interdisciplinary understanding.

Developing a standardized language to reflect the complexity and diversity of nursing practice is a challenging task. The language must represent patient experiences and be in a clinically useful form that is understandable to all members of the healthcare team. The North American Nursing Diagnosis Association (NANDA) believes its efforts contribute significantly to the accomplishment of that task. We are very pleased to present *NANDA Nursing Diagnoses: Definitions & Classification 2001–2002.* We think this edition clearly demonstrates NANDA's continuing effort to provide useful language to document the nurse's contribution to health care.

This edition has many features of previous editions; however, much has changed. Taxonomy II, presented to the membership at the 14th biennial conference in April 2000 and now the official taxonomic structure, is explained in detail. Consequently, the names of many of the diagnoses have changed. A list of the "old" and "new" diagnostic labels can be found in Table 1.1 on pages 3–10. In this book the names of the diagnoses are listed alphabetically by concept, which we believe will be clinically useful.

Seven new diagnoses are included in this edition. Sincere thanks go to the many nurses who took time from their busy professional lives to share these diagnoses with their colleagues. It takes dedication and effort to submit diagnoses for review, and NANDA is grateful. Nurses around the world will find documenting their practice is improved by the addition of these new diagnoses.

There are also six revised diagnoses. Although some revisions were submitted individually, the Nursing Diagnosis Extension Classification (NDEC) team from the University of Iowa undertook the majority of this work. NANDA is very grateful to all who submitted revisions. A dynamic nursing language is necessary if we hope to express the richness and change in nursing practices. Revisions always improve the specificity and sensitivity of the language.

In today's healthcare world where multiple systems must communicate across barriers of space, time, and technology, nurses need to use a standardized language. Without such a standardized language to represent nursing diagnoses, interventions, and outcomes, nursing cannot improve its ability to articulate its contributions to cost-effective, efficient, quality care. As efforts continue to develop reference terminologies to capture the whole healthcare experience, nursing must position itself to be a part of that development and must see that nursing is clearly represented in those terminologies. We believe this book contributes significantly to that effort.

Kay C. Avant, PhD, RN, FAAN
President, NANDA

New Nursing Diagnoses, April 2000

Risk for Falls
Risk for Powerlessness
Risk for Relocation Stress Syndrome
Risk for Situational Low Self-Esteem
Risk for Suicide
Self-Mutilation
Wandering

Introduction

Many things have changed in the last two years! The adoption of Taxonomy II required some significant modifications in the format of this book. Because NANDA seeks to assist clinicians, informaticists/system developers, and language developers alike, the NANDA board worked hard to come up with a format to serve everyone's needs efficiently. To make this book as user friendly as possible, but still useful to all three groups, it is divided into three parts.

Part 1 includes the traditional content of the previous *NANDA Nursing Diagnoses: Definitions & Classification* books and the nomenclature conversion table. A brief word of explanation may help you understand some of the changes in this section.

First, the nomenclature conversion table lists the diagnostic labels that were in Taxonomy I and the revised labels that are in Taxonomy II. You will note that several diagnoses have new modifiers (descriptors). This is because the NANDA Board of Directors asked the Taxonomy Committee to remove the word "altered" from the diagnostic modifiers. "Altered" means simply "changed," and does not give sufficient direction to clinicians who need to know more specifically *how or in what way* the phenomenon has been "altered." Thus, for example, you will find that "altered parenting" has become "impaired parenting." In each case the Taxonomy Committee used the defining characteristics of the diagnosis to choose a descriptor that most closely described the concept.

You will also note the diagnoses are listed in *alphabetical order by the diagnostic concept,* not by the first word or descriptor of the diagnosis. Taxonomy II splits the descriptors into axes (see Part 2, page 213, for a full explanation). Thus, if you are looking for "impaired wheelchair mobility," you will find it under "mobility," not under "wheelchair" or "impaired." We feel this will make the book much more clinically useful.

Part 2 introduces Taxonomy II, describes its structure and how it was developed, and provides two tables—Table 2.1, which explains the domains, classes, diagnostic concepts, and diagnoses; and Table 2.2, which shows the code conversions from Taxonomy I to Taxonomy II.

The conversion tables in Part 1 and Part 2 will help system developers adjust their systems to the new nomenclature and the new coding system. You will find these tables especially useful if you know the "old" name of the diagnosis and/or its placement in Taxonomy I but don't know whether its name has changed or in which domain it might be. If you are responsible for maintaining computerized patient records or your computer systems, you will need this code conversion table to help you in changing the codes from the old to the new taxonomy. The new coding system is not hierarchical as was the old one. The nonhierarchical coding allows us to add and subtract diagnoses without having to change the coding system again.

Part 3 contains diagnosis submission guidelines, diagnosis staging criteria, copyright guidelines; a list of members of the NANDA Board of Directors and the Taxonomy, Diagnosis Review, and NDEC Committees; and a glossary of terms.

How to Use This Book

The nursing diagnoses are listed alphabetically by *diagnostic concept*, which we believe will make this book very clinically useful. For example, *activity intolerance* is listed under "A" because activity is the diagnostic concept. Similarly, *interrupted family process* is listed under "F" because family process is the diagnostic concept. In Taxonomy II you will find that the names of many of the nursing diagnoses have been revised (see Table 1.1, Nomenclature Conversion, pp. 3–10).

We hope the organization of *NANDA Nursing Diagnoses: Definitions & Classification 2001–2001* will make it efficient and effective to use. We welcome your feedback. If you have suggestions, please send them to us through the NANDA Web site (http://www.nanda.org) or by calling the office at 800.647.9002.

Part 1

NANDA NURSING DIAGNOSES
2001–2002

The names and rules for naming (nomenclature) in Taxonomy II differ from those in Taxonomy I. In some diagnoses the wording was changed because of the multiaxial framework in Taxonomy II, and the Silver Ribbon Panel on Wellness recommended a new modifier for the wellness/health diagnoses "readiness for enhanced." Also, the NANDA Board of Directors deleted the term "altered" and added more descriptive terms (e.g., "impaired"). Finally, the Taxonomy Committee refined the rules for selection of modifiers to the nursing diagnoses so the selection would be in compliance with the new axial structure. The modifiers must be adjectives (see modifier definitions, page 219, to understand the changes). Table 1.1 shows the conversion from Taxonomy I wording to Taxonomy II wording.

Table 1.1   Nomenclature Conversion: Taxonomy I to Taxonomy II

Taxonomy I Nursing Diagnosis	*Taxonomy II Nursing Diagnosis*
Exchanging	
• Altered nutrition: More than body requirements	• Imbalanced nutrition: More than body requirements
• Altered nutrition: Less than body requirements	• Imbalanced nutrition: Less than body requirements
• Altered nutrition: Risk for more than body requirements	• Risk for imbalanced nutrition: More than body requirements
• Risk for infection	• Risk for infection
• Risk for altered body temperature	• Risk for imbalanced body temperature
• Hypothermia	• Hypothermia
• Hyperthermia	• Hyperthermia
• Ineffective thermoregulation	• Ineffective thermoregulation
• Dysreflexia	• Autonomic dysreflexia

continued

Table 1.1   Nomenclature Conversion   *continued*

Taxonomy I Nursing Diagnosis	*Taxonomy II Nursing Diagnosis*
• Risk for autonomic dysreflexia	• Risk for autonomic dysreflexia
• Constipation	• Constipation
• Perceived constipation	• Perceived constipation
• Diarrhea	• Diarrhea
• Bowel incontinence	• Bowel incontinence
• Risk for constipation	• Risk for constipation
• Altered urinary elimination	• Impaired urinary elimination
• Stress incontinence	• Stress urinary incontinence
• Reflex urinary incontinence	• Reflex urinary incontinence
• Urge incontinence	• Urge urinary incontinence
• Functional urinary incontinence	• Functional urinary incontinence
• Total incontinence	• Total urinary incontinence
• Risk for urinary urge incontinence	• Risk for urge urinary incontinence
• Urinary retention	• Urinary retention
• Altered tissue perfusion (specify type: renal, cerebral, cardio-pulmonary, gastrointestinal, peripheral)	• Ineffective tissue perfusion (specify type: renal, cerebral, cardiopulmonary, gastrointestinal, peripheral)
• Risk for fluid volume imbalance	• Risk for imbalanced fluid volume
• Fluid volume excess	• Excess fluid volume
• Fluid volume deficit	• Deficient fluid volume
• Risk for fluid volume deficit	• Risk for deficient fluid volume
• Decreased cardiac output	• Decreased cardiac output
• Impaired gas exchange	• Impaired gas exchange
• Ineffective airway clearance	• Ineffective airway clearance
• Ineffective breathing pattern	• Ineffective breathing pattern

Taxonomy I Nursing Diagnosis	**Taxonomy II Nursing Diagnosis**
• Inability to sustain spontaneous ventilation	• Impaired spontaneous ventilation
• Dysfunctional ventilatory weaning response	• Dysfunctional ventilatory weaning response
• Risk for injury	• Risk for injury
• Risk for suffocation	• Risk for suffocation
• Risk for poisoning	• Risk for poisoning
• Risk for trauma	• Risk for trauma
• Risk for aspiration	• Risk for aspiration
• Risk for disuse syndrome	• Risk for disuse syndrome
• Latex allergy response	• Latex allergy response
• Risk for latex allergy response	• Risk for latex allergy response
• Altered protection	• Ineffective protection
• Impaired tissue integrity	• Impaired tissue integrity
• Altered oral mucous membrane	• Impaired oral mucous membrane
• Impaired skin integrity	• Impaired skin integrity
• Risk for impaired skin integrity	• Risk for impaired skin integrity
• Altered dentition	• Impaired dentition
• Decreased adaptive capacity: Intracranial	• Decreased intracranial adaptive capacity
• Energy field disturbance	• Disturbed energy field
Communicating • Impaired verbal communication	• Impaired verbal communication
Relating • Impaired social interaction	• Impaired social interaction
• Social isolation	• Social isolation

continued

Table 1.1 Nomenclature Conversion *continued*

Taxonomy I Nursing Diagnosis	*Taxonomy II Nursing Diagnosis*
• Risk for loneliness	• Risk for loneliness
• Altered role performance	• Ineffective role performance
• Altered parenting	• Impaired parenting
• Risk for altered parenting	• Risk for impaired parenting
• Risk for altered parent/infant/child attachment	• Risk for impaired parent/infant/child attachment
• Sexual dysfunction	• Sexual dysfunction
• Altered family processes	• Interrupted family processes
• Caregiver role strain	• Caregiver role strain
• Risk for caregiver role strain	• Risk for caregiver role strain
• Altered family processes: Alcoholism	• Dysfunctional family processes: Alcoholism
• Parental role conflict	• Parental role conflict
• Altered sexuality patterns	• Ineffective sexuality patterns
Valuing	
• Spiritual distress (distress of the human spirit)	• Spiritual distress
• Risk for spiritual distress	• Risk for spiritual distress
• Potential for enhanced spiritual well-being	• Readiness for enhanced spiritual well-being
Choosing	
• Ineffective individual coping	• Ineffective coping
• Impaired adjustment	• Impaired adjustment
• Defensive coping	• Defensive coping
• Ineffective denial	• Ineffective denial
• Ineffective family coping: Disabling	• Disabled family coping

Taxonomy I Nursing Diagnosis	*Taxonomy II Nursing Diagnosis*
• Ineffective family coping: Compromised	• Compromised family coping
• Family coping: Potential for growth	• Readiness for enhanced family coping
• Potential for enhanced community coping	• Readiness for enhanced community coping
• Ineffective community coping	• Ineffective community coping
• Ineffective management of therapeutic regimen: Individual	• Ineffective therapeutic regimen management
• Noncompliance (specify)	• Noncompliance (specify)
• Ineffective management of therapeutic regimen: Families	• Ineffective family therapeutic regimen management
• Ineffective management of therapeutic regimen: Community	• Ineffective community therapeutic regimen management
• Effective management of therapeutic regimen: Individual	• Effective therapeutic regimen management
• Decisional conflict (specify)	• Decisional conflict (specify)
• Health-seeking behaviors (specify)	• Health-seeking behaviors (specify)

Moving

• Impaired physical mobility	• Impaired physical mobility
• Risk for peripheral neurovascular dysfunction	• Risk for peripheral neurovascular dysfunction
• Risk for perioperative-positioning injury	• Risk for perioperative-positioning injury
• Impaired walking	• Impaired walking
• Impaired wheelchair mobility	• Impaired wheelchair mobility
• Impaired transfer ability	• Impaired transfer ability

continued

Table 1.1 Nomenclature Conversion *continued*

Taxonomy I Nursing Diagnosis	*Taxonomy II Nursing Diagnosis*
• Impaired bed mobility	• Impaired bed mobility
• Activity intolerance	• Activity intolerance
• Fatigue	• Fatigue
• Risk for activity intolerance	• Risk for activity intolerance
• Sleep pattern disturbance	• Disturbed sleep pattern
• Sleep deprivation	• Sleep deprivation
• Diversional activity deficit	• Deficient diversional activity
• Impaired home maintenance management	• Impaired home maintenance
• Altered health maintenance	• Ineffective health maintenance
• Delayed surgical recovery	• Delayed surgical recovery
• Adult failure to thrive	• Adult failure to thrive
• Feeding self-care deficit	• Feeding self-care deficit
• Impaired swallowing	• Impaired swallowing
• Ineffective breastfeeding	• Ineffective breastfeeding
• Interrupted breastfeeding	• Interrupted breastfeeding
• Effective breastfeeding	• Effective breastfeeding
• Ineffective infant feeding pattern	• Ineffective infant feeding pattern
• Bathing/hygiene self-care deficit	• Bathing/hygiene self-care deficit
• Dressing/grooming self-care deficit	• Dressing/grooming self-care deficit
• Toileting self-care deficit	• Toileting self-care deficit
• Altered growth and development	• Delayed growth and development
• Risk for altered development	• Risk for delayed development
• Risk for altered growth	• Risk for disproportionate growth
• Relocation stress syndrome	• Relocation stress syndrome

Taxonomy I Nursing Diagnosis	*Taxonomy II Nursing Diagnosis*
• Risk for disorganized infant behavior	• Risk for disorganized infant behavior
• Disorganized infant behavior	• Disorganized infant behavior
• Potential for enhanced organized infant behavior	• Readiness for enhanced organized infant behavior

Perceiving

• Body image disturbance	• Disturbed body image
• Chronic low self-esteem	• Chronic low self-esteem
• Situational low self-esteem	• Situational low self-esteem
• Personal identity disturbance	• Disturbed personal identity
• Sensory/perceptual alterations (specify: visual, auditory, kinesthetic, gustatory, tactile, olfactory)	• Disturbed sensory perception (specify: visual, auditory, kinesthetic, gustatory, tactile, olfactory)
• Unilateral neglect	• Unilateral neglect
• Hopelessness	• Hopelessness
• Powerlessness	• Powerlessness

Knowing

• Knowledge deficit (specify)	• Deficient knowledge (specify)
• Impaired environmental-interpretation syndrome	• Impaired environmental interpretation syndrome
• Acute confusion	• Acute confusion
• Chronic confusion	• Chronic confusion
• Altered thought processes	• Disturbed thought processes
• Impaired memory	• Impaired memory

Feeling

• Pain	• Acute pain
• Chronic pain	• Chronic pain

continued

Table 1.1   Nomenclature Conversion *continued*

Taxonomy I Nursing Diagnosis	*Taxonomy II Nursing Diagnosis*
• Nausea	• Nausea
• Dysfunctional grieving	• Dysfunctional grieving
• Anticipatory grieving	• Anticipatory grieving
• Chronic sorrow	• Chronic sorrow
• Risk for violence: Directed at others	• Risk for other-directed violence
• Risk for self-mutilation	• Risk for self-mutilation
• Risk for violence: Self-directed	• Risk for self-directed violence
• Post-trauma syndrome	• Post-trauma syndrome
• Rape-trauma syndrome	• Rape-trauma syndrome
• Rape-trauma syndrome: Compound reaction	• Rape-trauma syndrome: Compound reaction
• Rape-trauma syndrome: Silent reaction	• Rape-trauma syndrome: Silent reaction
• Risk for post-trauma syndrome	• Risk for post-trauma syndrome
• Anxiety	• Anxiety
• Death anxiety	• Death anxiety
• Fear	• Fear
	New to Taxonomy II
	• Risk for falls
	• Risk for powerlessness
	• Risk for relocation stress syndrome
	• Risk for situational low self-esteem
	• Self-mutilation
	• Risk for suicide
	• Wandering

NANDA Nursing Diagnoses
With Definitions,
Defining Characteristics or
Risk Factors, and Related Factors

ACTIVITY INTOLERANCE
(1982)

Definition *Insufficient physiological or psychological energy to endure or complete required or desired daily activities*

Defining Characteristics
- Verbal report of fatigue or weakness
- Abnormal heart rate or blood pressure response to activity
- Electrocardiographic changes reflecting arrhythmias or ischemia
- Exertional discomfort or dyspnea

Related Factors
Bed rest or immobility
Generalized weakness
Imbalance between oxygen supply/demand
Sedentary lifestyle

RISK FOR ACTIVITY INTOLERANCE
(1982)

Definition *At risk for experiencing insufficient physiological or psychological energy to endure or complete required or desired daily activities*

Risk Factors

Inexperience with the
activity
Presence of circulatory/
respiratory problems
History of previous
intolerance
Deconditioned status

IMPAIRED ADJUSTMENT
(1986, 1998)

Definition   *Inability to modify lifestyle/behavior in a manner consistent with a change in health status*

Defining Characteristics

- Denial of health status change
- Failure to take actions that would prevent further health problems
- Failure to achieve optimal sense of control
- Demonstration of nonacceptance of health status change

Related Factors

Low state of optimism
Intense emotional state
Negative attitudes toward health behavior
Absence of intent to change behavior
Multiple stressors
Absence of social support for changed beliefs and practices

Disability or health status change requiring change in lifestyle
Lack of motivation to change behaviors

INEFFECTIVE AIRWAY CLEARANCE
(1980, 1996, 1998)

Definition *Inability to clear secretions or obstructions from the respiratory tract to maintain a clear airway*

Defining Characteristics

- Dyspnea
- Diminished breath sounds
- Orthopnea
- Adventitious breath sounds (rales, crackles, rhonchi, wheezes)
- Cough, ineffective or absent
- Sputum production
- Cyanosis
- Difficulty vocalizing
- Wide-eyed
- Changes in respiratory rate and rhythm
- Restlessness

Related Factors

Environmental

Smoking
Smoke inhalation
Second-hand smoke

Obstructed airway

Airway spasm
Retained secretions
Excessive mucus
Presence of artificial airway
Foreign body in airway
Secretions in the bronchi
Exudate in the alveoli

Physiological

Neuromuscular dysfunction
Hyperplasia of the bronchial walls
Chronic obstructive pulmonary disease
Infection
Asthma
Allergic airways

LATEX ALLERGY RESPONSE
(1998)

Definition *An allergic response to natural latex rubber products*

Defining Characteristics

Type I Reactions

- Immediate reactions (<1 hour) to latex proteins (can be life threatening)
- Contact urticaria progressing to generalized symptoms
- Edema of the lips, tongue, uvula, and/or throat
- Shortness of breath, tightness in chest, wheezing, bronchospasm leading to respiratory arrest
- Hypotension, syncope, cardiac arrest

May also include:

- Orofacial characteristics
  - Edema of sclera or eyelids
  - Erythema and/or itching of the eyes
  - Tearing of the eyes
  - Nasal congestion, itching, and/or erythema
  - Rhinorrhea
  - Facial erythema
  - Facial itching
  - Oral itching
- Gastrointestinal characteristics
  - Abdominal pain
  - Nausea
- Generalized characteristics
  - Flushing
  - General discomfort
  - Generalized edema
  - Increasing complaint of total body warmth
  - Restlessness

Type IV Reactions

- Delayed onset (hours)
- Eczema
- Irritation
- Reaction to additives (e.g., thiurams, carbamates) causes discomfort
- Redness

Irritant Reactions

- Erythema
- Chapped or cracked skin
- Blisters

Related Factors

No immune mechanism response

RISK FOR LATEX ALLERGY RESPONSE
(1998)

Definition *At risk for allergic response to natural latex rubber products*

Risk Factors

Multiple surgical procedures, especially from infancy (e.g., spina bifida)

Allergies to bananas, avocados, tropical fruits, kiwi, chestnuts

Professions with daily exposure to latex (e.g., medicine, nursing, dentistry)

Conditions associated with continuous or intermittent catheterization

History of reactions to latex (e.g., balloons, condoms, gloves)

Allergies to poinsettia plants

History of allergies and asthma

ANXIETY
(1973, 1982, 1998)

Definition   *Vague uneasy feeling of discomfort or dread accompanied by an autonomic response (the source often non-specific or unknown to the individual); a feeling of apprehension caused by anticipation of danger. It is an alerting signal that warns of impending danger and enables the individual to take measures to deal with threat.*

Defining Characteristics

Behavioral
- Diminished productivity
- Scanning and vigilance
- Poor eye contact
- Restlessness
- Glancing about
- Extraneous movement (e.g., foot shuffling, hand/arm movements)
- Expressed concerns due to change in life events
- Insomnia
- Fidgeting

Affective
- Regretful
- Irritability
- Anguish
- Scared
- Jittery
- Overexcited
- Painful and persistent increased helplessness
- Rattled
- Uncertainty
- Increased wariness

- Focus on self
- Feelings of inadequacy
- Fearful
- Distressed
- Worried, apprehensive
- Anxious

Physiological
- Voice quivering
- Trembling/hand tremors
- Shakiness
- Increased respiration (sympathetic)
- Urinary urgency (parasympathetic)
- Increased pulse (sympathetic)
- Pupil dilation (sympathetic)
- Increased reflexes (sympathetic)
- Abdominal pain (parasympathetic)
- Sleep disturbance (parasympathetic)

continued

Anxiety, *continued*

- Tingling in extremities (parasympathetic)
- Cardiovascular excitation (sympathetic)
- Increased perspiration
- Facial tension
- Anorexia (sympathetic)
- Heart pounding (sympathetic)
- Diarrhea (parasympathetic)
- Urinary hesitancy (parasympathetic)
- Fatigue (parasympathetic)
- Dry mouth (sympathetic)
- Weakness (sympathetic)
- Decreased pulse (parasympathetic)
- Facial flushing (sympathetic)
- Superficial vasoconstriction (sympathetic)
- Twitching (sympathetic)
- Decreased blood pressure (parasympathetic)
- Nausea (parasympathetic)
- Urinary frequency (parasympathetic)
- Faintness (parasympathetic)
- Respiratory difficulties (sympathetic)
- Increased blood pressure (sympathetic)

Cognitive

- Blocking of thought
- Confusion
- Preoccupation
- Forgetfulness
- Rumination
- Impaired attention
- Decreased perceptual field
- Fear of unspecified consequences
- Tendency to blame others
- Difficulty concentrating
- Diminished ability to
  – Problem solve
  – Learn
- Awareness of physiologic symptoms

Related Factors

Exposure to toxins
Unconscious conflict
  about essential
  values/goals of life
Familial association/
  heredity
Unmet needs
Interpersonal
  transmission/contagion
Situational/maturational
  crises
Threat of death

Threat to self-concept
Stress
Substance abuse
Threat to or change in
– Role status
– Health status
– Interaction patterns
– Role function
– Environment
– Economic status

DEATH ANXIETY
(1998)

Definition *Apprehension, worry, or fear related to death or dying*

Defining Characteristics

- Worrying about the impact of one's own death on significant others
- Powerless over issues related to dying
- Fear of loss of physical and/or mental abilities when dying
- Anticipated pain related to dying
- Deep sadness
- Fear of the process of dying
- Concerns of overworking the caregiver as terminal illness incapacitates self
- Concern about meeting one's creator or feeling doubtful about the existence of a God or Higher Being

- Total loss of control over any aspect of one's own death
- Negative death images or unpleasant thoughts about any event related to death or dying
- Fear of delayed demise
- Fear of premature death because it prevents the accomplishment of important life goals
- Worrying about being the cause of other's grief and suffering
- Fear of leaving family alone after death
- Fear of developing a terminal illness
- Denial of one's own mortality or impending death

Related Factors

To be developed

RISK FOR ASPIRATION
(1988)

Definition   *At risk for entry of gastrointestinal secretions, oropharyngeal secretions, solids, or fluids into tracheobronchial passages*

Risk Factors

Increased intragastric pressure
Tube feedings
Situations hindering elevation of upper body
Reduced level of consciousness
Presence of tracheostomy or endotracheal tube
Medication administration
Wired jaws
Increased gastric residual

Incompetent lower esophageal sphincter
Impaired swallowing
Gastrointestinal tubes
Facial, oral, neck surgery or trauma
Depressed cough and gag reflexes
Decreased gastrointestinal motility
Delayed gastric emptying

RISK FOR IMPAIRED PARENT/INFANT/ CHILD ATTACHMENT*
(1994)

Definition *Disruption of the interactive process between parent/significant other and infant that fosters the development of a protective and nurturing reciprocal relationship*

Risk Factors

Physical barriers
Anxiety associated with the parent role
Substance abuse
Premature infant, ill infant/child who is unable to effectively initiate parental contact due to altered behavioral organization

Lack of privacy
Inability of parents to meet personal needs
Separation

---

* Formerly "Risk for Altered Parent/Infant-Child Attachment"

Autonomic Dysreflexia*
(1988)

Definition *Life-threatening, uninhibited sympathetic response of the nervous system to a noxious stimulus after a spinal cord injury at T7 or above*

Defining Characteristics

- Pallor (below the injury)
- Paroxysmal hypertension (sudden periodic elevated blood pressure with systolic pressure >140 mm Hg and diastolic pressure >90 mm Hg)
- Red splotches on skin (above the injury)
- Bradycardia or tachycardia (heart rate <60 or >100 beats per minute)
- Diaphoresis (above the injury)
- Headache (a diffuse pain in different portions of the head and not confined to any nerve distribution area)
- Blurred vision
- Chest pain
- Chilling
- Conjunctival congestion
- Horner's syndrome (contraction of the pupil, partial ptosis of the eyelid, enophthalmos and sometimes loss of sweating over the affected side of the face)
- Metallic taste in mouth
- Nasal congestion
- Paresthesia
- Pilomotor reflex (gooseflesh formation when skin is cooled)

Related Factors

Bladder distention
Bowel distention
Lack of patient and
  caregiver knowledge
Skin irritation

* *Formerly "Dysreflexia"*

RISK FOR AUTONOMIC DYSREFLEXIA
(1998, 2000)

Definition *At risk for life-threatening, uninhibited response of the sympathetic nervous system, post spinal shock, in an individual with spinal cord injury or lesion at T6 or above (has been demonstrated in patients with injuries at T7 and T8)*

Defining Characteristics

An injury/lesion at T6 or above AND at least one of the following noxious stimuli:

Neurological Stimuli
- Painful/irritating stimuli below level of injury

Urological Stimuli
- Bladder distention
- Detrusor sphincter dyssynergia
- Bladder spasm
- Instrumentation or surgery
- Epididymitis
- Urethritis
- Urinary tract infection
- Calculi
- Cystitis
- Catheterization

Gastrointestinal Stimuli
- Bowel distention
- Fecal impaction
- Digital stimulation
- Suppositories
- Hemorrhoids
- Difficult passage of feces
- Constipation
- Enemas
- GI system pathology
- Gastric ulcers
- Esophageal reflux
- Gallstones

Reproductive Stimuli
- Menstruation
- Sexual intercourse
- Pregnancy
- Labor and delivery
- Ovarian cyst
- Ejaculation

Musculo-Skeletal-Integumentary Stimuli
- Cutaneous stimulation (e.g., pressure ulcer, ingrown toenail, dressings, burns, rash)
- Pressure over bony prominences or genitalia
- Heterotrophic bone
- Spasm
- Fractures
- Range-of-motion exercises

- Wounds
- Sunburns

Regulatory Stimuli

- Temperature fluctuations
- Extreme environmental temperatures

Situational Stimuli

- Positioning
- Constrictive clothing (e.g., straps, stockings, shoes)

- Drug reactions (e.g., decongestants, sympathomimetics, vasoconstrictors, narcotic withdrawal)
- Surgical procedure

Cardiac/Pulmonary Problems

- Pulmonary emboli
- Deep vein thrombosis

DISTURBED BODY IMAGE*
(1973, 1998)

Definition *Confusion in mental picture of one's physical self*

Defining Characteristics

- Verbalization of feelings that reflect an altered view of one's body in appearance, structure, or function
- Verbalization of perceptions that reflect an altered view of one's body in appearance, structure, or function
- Nonverbal response to actual or perceived change in body structure and/or function
- Behaviors of avoidance, monitoring, or acknowledgment of one's body

Objective

- Missing body part
- Trauma to nonfunctioning part
- Not touching body part
- Hiding or overexposing body part (intentional or unintentional)

- Actual change in structure and/or function
- Change in social involvement
- Change in ability to estimate spatial relationship of body to environment
- Extension of body boundary to incorporate environmental objects
- Not looking at body part

Subjective

- Refusal to verify actual change
- Preoccupation with change or loss
- Personalization of part or loss by name
- Depersonalization of part or loss by impersonal pronouns
- Extension of body boundary to incorporate environmental objects

---

* *Formerly "Body Image Disturbance"*

B

- Negative feelings about body (e.g., feelings of helplessness, hopelessness, or powerlessness)
- Verbalization of change in lifestyle
- Focus on past strength, function, or appearance

- Fear of rejection or of reaction by others
- Emphasis on remaining strengths
- Heightened achievement

Related Factors

Psychosocial
Biophysical
Cognitive/perceptual
Cultural or spiritual
Developmental changes

Illness
Trauma or injury
Surgery
Illness treatment

B

RISK FOR IMBALANCED Body TEMPERATURE*
(1986)

Definition *At risk for failure to maintain body temperature within normal range*

Risk Factors

Altered metabolic rate

Illness or trauma affecting temperature regulation

Medications causing vasoconstriction or vasodilation

Inappropriate clothing for environmental temperature

Inactivity or vigorous activity

Extremes of weight

Extremes of age

Dehydration

Sedation

Exposure to cold/cool or warm/hot environments

* Formerly "Risk for Altered Body Temperature"

Bowel Incontinence
(1975, 1998)

Definition *Change in normal bowel habits characterized by involuntary passage of stool*

Defining Characteristics

- Constant dribbling of soft stool
- Fecal odor
- Inability to delay defecation
- Urgency
- Self-report of inability to feel rectal fullness
- Fecal staining of clothing and/or bedding
- Recognizes rectal fullness but reports inability to expel formed stool
- Inattention to urge to defecate
- Inability to recognize urge to defecate
- Red perianal skin

Related Factors

Environmental factors (e.g., inaccessible bathroom)
Incomplete emptying of bowel
Rectal sphincter abnormality
Impaction
Dietary habits
Colorectal lesions
Stress
Lower motor nerve damage
Abnormally high abdominal or intestinal pressure
General decline in muscle tone
Loss of rectal sphincter control
Impaired cognition
Upper motor nerve damage
Chronic diarrhea
Toileting self-care deficit
Impaired reservoir capacity
Medications
Immobility
Laxative abuse

B

EFFECTIVE BREASTFEEDING
(1990)

Definition *Mother-infant dyad/family exhibits adequate proficiency and satisfaction with breastfeeding process*

Defining Characteristics

- Effective mother/infant communication patterns
- Regular and sustained suckling/swallowing at the breast
- Appropriate infant weight pattern for age
- Infant content after feeding
- Mother able to position infant at breast to promote a successful latch-on response
- Signs and/or symptoms of oxytocin release
- Adequate infant elimination patterns for age
- Eagerness of infant to nurse
- Maternal verbalization of satisfaction with the breastfeeding process

Related Factors

Infant gestational age >34 weeks
Support source
Normal infant oral structure
Maternal confidence
Basic breastfeeding knowledge
Normal breast structure

INEFFECTIVE BREASTFEEDING
(1988)

Definition *Dissatisfaction or difficulty a mother, infant, or child experiences with the breastfeeding process*

Defining Characteristics

- Unsatisfactory breast-feeding process
- Nonsustained suckling at the breast
- Resisting latching on
- Unresponsive to comfort measures
- Persistence of sore nipples beyond first week of breastfeeding
- Observable signs of inadequate infant intake
- Insufficient emptying of each breast per feeding
- Infant inability to attach on to maternal breast correctly

- Infant arching and crying at the breast
- Infant exhibiting fussiness and crying within the first hour after breastfeeding
- Actual or perceived inadequate milk supply
- No observable signs of oxytocin release
- Insufficient opportunity for suckling at the breast

Related Factors

Nonsupportive partner/ family
Previous breast surgery
Infant receiving supplemental feedings with artificial nipple
Prematurity
Previous history of breastfeeding failure

Poor infant sucking reflex
Maternal breast anomaly
Maternal anxiety or ambivalence
Interruption in breastfeeding
Infant anomaly
Knowledge deficit

B

INTERRUPTED BREASTFEEDING
(1992)

Definition   *Break in the continuity of the breastfeeding process as a result of inability or inadvisability to put baby to breast for feeding*

Defining Characteristics

- Infant receives no nourishment at the breast for some or all of feedings
- Maternal desire to maintain and provide (or eventually provide) her breast milk for her infant's nutritional needs
- Lack of knowledge regarding expression and storage of breast milk
- Separation of mother and infant

Related Factors

Contraindications to breastfeeding
Maternal employment
Maternal or infant illness
Need to abruptly wean infant
Prematurity

INEFFECTIVE BREATHING PATTERN
(1980, 1996, 1998)

Definition *Inspiration and/or expiration that does not provide adequate ventilation*

Defining Characteristics

- Decreased inspiratory/ expiratory pressure
- Decreased minute ventilation
- Use of accessory muscles to breathe
- Nasal flaring
- Dyspnea
- Orthopnea
- Altered chest excursion
- Shortness of breath
- Assumption of 3-point position
- Pursed-lip breathing
- Prolonged expiration phases
- Increased anterior-posterior diameter
- Respiratory rate/min:
  - Infants: <25 or >60
  - Ages 1–4: <20 or >30
  - Ages 5–14: <14 or >25
  - Adults >14: ≤11 or >24
- Depth of breathing
  - Adult tidal volume: 500 ml at rest
  - Infant tidal volume: 6–8 ml/Kg
- Timing ratio
- Decreased vital capacity

Related Factors

Hyperventilation
Hypoventilation syndrome
Bony deformity
Pain
Chest wall deformity
Anxiety
Decreased energy/ fatigue
Neuromuscular dysfunction
Musculoskeletal impairment
Perception/cognitive impairment
Obesity
Spinal cord injury
Body position
Neurological immaturity
Respiratory muscle fatigue

C **C**

DECREASED CARDIAC OUTPUT
(1975, 1996, 2000)

Definition *Inadequate blood pumped by the heart to meet metabolic demands of the body*

Defining Characteristics

Altered Heart Rate/ Rhythm

- Arrhythmias (tachycardia, bradycardia)
- Palpitations
- EKG changes

Altered Preload

- Jugular vein distention
- Fatigue
- Edema
- Murmurs
- Increased/decreased central venous pressure (CVP)
- Increased/decreased pulmonary artery wedge pressure (PAWP)
- Weight gain

Altered Afterload

- Cold/clammy skin
- Shortness of breath/ dyspnea
- Oliguria
- Prolonged capillary refill
- Decreased peripheral pulses

- Variations in blood pressure readings
- Increased/decreased systemic vascular resistance (SVR)
- Increased/decreased pulmonary vascular resistance (PVR)
- Skin color changes

Altered Contractility

- Crackles
- Cough
- Orthopnea/paroxysmal nocturnal dyspnea
- Cardiac output <4 L/min
- Cardiac index <2.5 L/min
- Decreased ejection fraction, Stroke Volume Index (SVI), Left Ventricular Stroke Work Index (LVSWI)
- S3 or S4 sounds

Behavioral/Emotional

- Anxiety
- Restlessness

Related Factors

Altered heart rate/
  rhythm

Altered Stroke Volume

Altered preload
Altered afterload
Altered contractility

C

C CAREGIVER ROLE STRAIN
(1992, 1998, 2000)

Definition *Difficulty in performing caregiver role*

Defining Characteristics

Caregiving Activities

- Difficulty performing/completing required tasks
- Preoccupation with care routine
- Apprehension about the future regarding care receiver's health and the caregiver's ability to provide care
- Apprehension about care receiver's care if caregiver becomes ill or dies
- Dysfunctional change in caregiving activities
- Apprehension about possible institutionalization of care receiver

Caregiver Health Status

Physical

- GI upset (e.g., mild stomach cramps, vomiting, diarrhea, recurrent gastric ulcer episodes)
- Weight change
- Rash
- Hypertension
- Cardiovascular disease
- Diabetes
- Fatigue
- Headaches

Emotional

- Impaired individual coping
- Feeling depressed
- Disturbed sleep
- Anger
- Stress
- Somatization
- Increased nervousness
- Increased emotional lability
- Impatience
- Lack of time to meet personal needs
- Frustration

Socioeconomic

- Withdraws from social life
- Changes in leisure activities
- Low work productivity
- Refuses career advancement

C

Caregiver-Care Receiver Relationship
- Grief/uncertainty regarding changed relationship with care receiver
- Difficulty watching care receiver go through the illness

Family Processes
- Family conflict
- Concerns about family members

Related Factors

Care Receiver Health Status

Illness severity
Illness chronicity
Increasing care needs/dependency
Unpredictability of illness course
Instability of care receiver's health
Problem behaviors
Psychological or cognitive problems
Addiction or codependency

Caregiving Activities

Amount of activities
Complexity of activities
24-hour care responsibilities
Ongoing changes in activities
Discharge of family members to home with significant care needs

Years of caregiving
Unpredictability of care situation

Caregiver Health Status

Physical problems
Psychological or cognitive problems
Addiction or codependency
Marginal coping patterns
Unrealistic expectations of self
Inability to fulfill one's own or other's expectations

Socioeconomic

Isolation from others
Competing role commitments
Alienation from family, friends, and co-workers
Insufficient recreation

continued

Caregiver Role Strain, *continued*

Caregiver-Care Receiver Relationship

History of poor relationship

Presence of abuse or violence

Unrealistic expectations of caregiver by care receiver

Mental status of elder inhibiting conversation

Family Processes

History of marginal family coping

History of family dysfunction

Resources

Inadequate physical environment for providing care (e.g., housing, temperature, safety)

Inadequate equipment for providing care

Inadequate transportation

Inadequate community resources (e.g., respite services, recreational resources)

Insufficient finances

Lack of support

Caregiver is not developmentally ready for caregiver role

Inexperience with caregiving

Insufficient time

Lack of knowledge about or difficulty accessing community resources

Lack of caregiver privacy

Emotional strength

Physical energy

Assistance and support (formal and informal)

RISK FOR CAREGIVER ROLE STRAIN
(1992)

C

Definition   *Caregiver is vulnerable for felt difficulty in performing the family caregiver role*

Risk Factors

Caregiver not developmentally ready for caregiver role (e.g., a young adult needing to provide care for middle aged)

Inadequate physical environment for providing care (e.g., housing, transportation, community services, equipment)

Unpredictable illness course or instability in the care receiver's health

Psychological or cognitive problems in care receiver

Presence of situational stressors that normally affect families (e.g., significant loss, disaster or crisis, economic vulnerability, major life events)

Presence of abuse or violence

Premature birth/congenital defect

Past history of poor relationship between caregiver and care receiver

Marginal family adaptation or dysfunction prior to the caregiving situation

Marginal caregiver's coping patterns

Lack of respite and recreation for caregiver

Inexperience with caregiving

Caregiver is female

Addiction or codependency

Care receiver exhibits deviant, bizarre behavior

Caregiver's competing role commitments

Caregiver health impairment

Illness severity of the care receiver

Caregiver is spouse

Developmental delay or retardation of the care receiver or caregiver

continued

Risk for Caregiver Role Strain, *continued*

C

Complexity/amount of
  caregiving tasks
Discharge of family
  member with significant
  home care needs
Duration of caregiving
  required
Family/caregiver isolation

IMPAIRED VERBAL COMMUNICATION
(1983, 1996, 1998)

C

Definition   *Decreased, delayed, or absent ability to receive, process, transmit, and use a system of symbols*

Defining Characteristics

- Willful refusal to speak
- Disorientation in the three spheres of time, space, person
- Inability to speak dominant language
- Does not or cannot speak
- Speaks or verbalizes with difficulty
- Inappropriate verbalization
- Difficulty forming words or sentences (e.g., aphonia, dyslalia, dysarthria)
- Difficulty expressing thought verbally (e.g., aphasia, dysphasia, apraxia, dyslexia)
- Stuttering
- Slurring
- Dyspnea
- Absence of eye contact or difficulty in selective attending
- Difficulty in comprehending and maintaining usual communication pattern
- Partial or total visual deficit
- Inability or difficulty in use of facial or body expressions

Related Factors

Decrease in circulation to brain
Cultural difference
Psychological barriers (e.g., psychosis, lack of stimuli)
Physical barrier (tracheostomy, intubation)
Anatomical defect (e.g., cleft palate, alteration of the neuromuscular visual system, auditory system, phonatory apparatus)
Brain tumor

continued

Impaired Verbal Communication, *continued*

C

Differences related to developmental age
Side effects of medication
Environmental barriers
Absence of significant others
Altered perceptions
Lack of information
Stress
Alteration of self-esteem or self-concept
Physiological conditions
Alteration of central nervous system
Weakening of the musculoskeletal system
Emotional conditions

DECISIONAL CONFLICT (Specify)
(1988)

Definition   *Uncertainty about course of action to be taken when choice among competing actions involves risk, loss, or challenge to personal life values*

Defining Characteristics

- Verbalizes uncertainty about choices
- Verbalizes undesired consequences of alternative actions being considered
- Vacillation between alternative choices
- Delayed decision making
- Verbalizes feeling of distress while attempting a decision
- Self-focusing
- Physical signs of distress or tension (e.g., increased heart rate, increased muscle tension, restlessness)
- Questioning personal values and beliefs while attempting a decision

Related Factors

Support system deficit
Perceived threat to value system
Lack of experience or interference with decision making

Multiple or divergent sources of information
Lack of relevant information
Unclear personal values/ beliefs

C

PARENTAL ROLE Conflict
(1988)

Definition *Parent experience of role confusion and conflict in response to crisis*

Defining Characteristics

- Parent(s) express(es) concern(s) about changes in parental role, family functioning, family communication, family health
- Parent(s) express(es) concern(s)/feeling(s) of inadequacy to provide for child's physical and emotional needs during hospitalization or in home
- Reluctant to participate in usual caretaking activities even with encouragement and support

- Demonstrated disruption in caretaking routines
- Expresses concern about perceived loss of control over decisions relating to their child
- Verbalizes or demonstrates feelings of guilt, anger, fear, anxiety, and/or frustrations about effect of child's illness on family process

Related Factors

Change in marital status
Home care of a child with special needs (e.g., apnea monitoring, postural drainage, hyperalimentation)
Interruptions of family life due to home care regimen (e.g., treatments, caregivers, lack of respite)

Specialized care-center policies
Separation from child due to chronic illness
Intimidation with invasive or restrictive modalities (e.g., isolation, intubation)

ACUTE CONFUSION
(1994)

Definition *Abrupt onset of a cluster of global, transient changes and disturbances in attention, cognition, psychomotor activity, level of consciousness, and/or sleep/wake cycle*

Defining Characteristics

- Lack of motivation to initiate and/or follow through with goal-directed or purposeful behavior
- Fluctuation in psychomotor activity
- Misperceptions
- Fluctuation in cognition
- Increased agitation or restlessness
- Fluctuation in level of consciousness
- Fluctuation in sleep-wake cycle
- Hallucinations

Related Factors

Over 60 years of age
Alcohol abuse
Delirium
Dementia
Drug abuse

C

CHRONIC CONFUSION
(1994)

Definition   *Irreversible, long-standing, and/or progressive deterioration of intellect and personality characterized by decreased ability to interpret environmental stimuli; decreased capacity for intellectual thought processes; and manifested by disturbances of memory, orientation, and behavior*

Defining Characteristics
- Altered interpretation/ response to stimuli
- Clinical evidence of organic impairment
- Progressive/long-standing cognitive impairment
- Altered personality
- Impaired memory (short- and long-term)
- Impaired socialization
- No change in level of consciousness

Related Factors
Multi-infarct dementia
Korsakoff's psychosis
Head injury
Alzheimer's disease
Cerebral vascular accident

Constipation
(1975, 1998)

Definition   *Decrease in normal frequency of defecation accompanied by difficult or incomplete passage of stool and/or passage of excessively hard, dry stool*

Defining Characteristics

- Change in bowel pattern
- Bright red blood with stool
- Presence of soft, pastelike stool in rectum
- Distended abdomen
- Dark, black, or tarry stool
- Increased abdominal pressure
- Percussed abdominal dullness
- Pain with defecation
- Decreased volume of stool
- Straining with defecation
- Decreased frequency
- Dry, hard, formed stool
- Palpable rectal mass
- Feeling of rectal fullness or pressure
- Abdominal pain
- Unable to pass stool
- Anorexia
- Headache
- Change in abdominal growling (borborygmi)
- Indigestion
- Atypical presentations in older adults (e.g., change in mental status, urinary incontinence, unexplained falls, elevated body temperature)
- Severe flatus
- Generalized fatigue
- Hypoactive or hyperactive bowel sounds
- Palpable abdominal mass
- Abdominal tenderness with or without palpable muscle resistance
- Nausea and/or vomiting
- Oozing liquid stool

continued

C

Constipation, *continued*

Related Factors

Functional

Recent environmental
changes
Habitual denial/ignoring
of urge to defecate
Insufficient physical
activity
Irregular defecation
habits
Inadequate toileting (e.g.,
timeliness, positioning
for defecation, privacy)
Abdominal muscle
weakness

Psychological

Depression
Emotional stress
Mental confusion

Pharmacological

Anticonvulsants
Antilipemic agents
Laxative overdose
Calcium carbonate
Aluminum-containing
antacids
Nonsteroidal anti-
inflammatory agents
Opiates
Anticholinergics
Diuretics
Iron salts
Phenothiazines
Sedatives
Sympathomimetics
Bismuth salts
Antidepressants
Calcium channel blockers

Mechanical

Rectal abscess or ulcer
Pregnancy
Rectal anal fissures
Tumors
Megacolon
(Hirschsprung's disease)
Electrolyte imbalance
Rectal prolapse
Prostate enlargement
Neurological impairment
Rectal anal stricture
Rectocele
Postsurgical obstruction
Hemorrhoids
Obesity

Physiological

Poor eating habits
Decreased motility of
gastrointestinal tract
Inadequate dentition or
oral hygiene
Insufficient fiber intake
Insufficient fluid intake
Change in usual foods
and eating patterns
Dehydration

PERCEIVED CONSTIPATION
(1988)

C

Definition *Self-diagnosis of constipation and abuse of laxatives, enemas, and suppositories to ensure a daily bowel movement*

Defining Characteristics

- Expectation of a daily bowel movement with resulting overuse of laxatives, enemas, and suppositories
- Expectation of passage of stool at same time every day

Related Factors

Impaired thought processes
Faulty appraisal
Cultural/family health beliefs

C RISK FOR CONSTIPATION
(1998)

Definition *At risk for a decrease in normal frequency of defecation accompanied by difficult or incomplete passage of stool and/or passage of excessively hard, dry stool*

Risk Factors

Functional

Habitual denial/ignoring of urge to defecate
Recent environmental changes
Inadequate toileting (e.g., timeliness, positioning for defecation, privacy)
Irregular defecation habits
Insufficient physical activity
Abdominal muscle weakness

Psychological

Emotional stress
Mental confusion
Depression

Physiological

Insufficient fiber intake
Dehydration
Inadequate dentition or oral hygiene
Poor eating habits
Insufficient fluid intake
Change in usual foods and eating patterns
Decreased motility of gastrointestinal tract

Pharmacological

Anticonvulsants
Phenothiazines
Nonsteroidal anti-inflammatory agents
Sedatives
Aluminum-containing antacids
Laxative overuse
Iron salts
Anticholinergics
Antidepressants
Antilipemic agents
Calcium channel blockers
Calcium carbonate
Diuretics
Sympathomimetics
Opiates
Bismuth salts

Mechanical

Rectal abscess or ulcer
Pregnancy
Rectal anal stricture
Postsurgical obstruction
Rectal anal fissures
Megacolon (Hirschsprung's disease)
Electrolyte imbalance

Tumors
Prostate enlargement
Rectocele
Rectal prolapse
Neurological impairment
Hemorrhoids
Obesity

C

C

INEFFECTIVE COPING
(1978, 1998)

Definition *Inability to form a valid appraisal of the stressors, inadequate choices of practiced responses, and/or inability to use available resources*

Defining Characteristics

- Lack of goal-directed behavior/resolution of problem, including inability to attend to and difficulty organizing information
- Sleep disturbance
- Abuse of chemical agents
- Decreased use of social support
- Use of forms of coping that impede adaptive behavior
- Poor concentration
- Fatigue
- Inadequate problem solving
- Verbalization of inability to cope or inability to ask for help
- Inability to meet basic needs
- Destructive behavior toward self or others
- Inability to meet role expectations
- High illness rate
- Change in usual communication patterns
- Risk taking

Related Factors

Gender differences in coping strategies
Inadequate level of confidence in ability to cope
Uncertainty
Inadequate social support created by characteristics of relationships
Inadequate level of perception of control
Inadequate resources available

High degree of threat
Situational or maturational crisis
Disturbance in pattern of tension release
Inadequate opportunity to prepare for stressor
Inability to conserve adaptive energies
Disturbance in pattern of appraisal of threat

INEFFECTIVE COMMUNITY COPING
(1994, 1998)

C

Definition *Pattern of community activities (for adaptation and problem solving) that is unsatisfactory for meeting the demands or needs of the community*

Defining Characteristics

- Expressed community powerlessness
- Deficits in community participation
- Excessive community conflicts
- Expressed vulnerability
- High illness rates
- Stressors perceived as excessive
- Community does not meet its own expectations
- Increased social problems (e.g., homicides, vandalism, arson, terrorism, robbery, infanticide, abuse, divorce, unemployment, poverty, militancy, mental illness)

Related Factors

Natural or man-made disasters

Ineffective or nonexistent community systems (e.g., lack of emergency medical system, transportation system, or disaster planning systems)

Deficits in community social support services and resources

Inadequate resources for problem solving

C

READINESS FOR ENHANCED COMMUNITY COPING*
(1994)

Definition *Pattern of community activities for adaptation and problem solving that is satisfactory for meeting the demands or needs of the community but can be improved for management of current and future problems/stressors*

Defining Characteristics

- One or more characteristics that indicate effective coping:
  - Positive communication between community/aggregates and larger community
  - Programs available for recreation and relaxation
  - Resources sufficient for managing stressors
  - Agreement that community is responsible for stress management
  - Active planning by community for predicted stressors
  - Active problem solving by community when faced with issues
  - Positive communication among community members

Related Factors

Community has a sense of power to manage stressors

Social supports available

Resources available for problem solving

* *Formerly "Potential for Enhanced Community Coping"*

DEFENSIVE COPING
(1988)

Definition *Repeated projection of falsely positive self-evaluation based on a self-protective pattern that defends against underlying perceived threats to positive self-regard*

Defining Characteristics

- Grandiosity
- Rationalization of failures
- Hypersensitivity to slight/criticism
- Denial of obvious problems/weaknesses
- Projection of blame/responsibility
- Lack of follow-through or participation in treatment or therapy
- Superior attitude toward others
- Hostile laughter or ridicule of others
- Difficulty in perception of reality/reality testing
- Difficulty establishing/maintaining relationships

Related Factors

To be developed

C

COMPROMISED FAMILY COPING*
(1980, 1996)

Definition   *Usually supportive primary person (family member or close friend) provides insufficient, ineffective, or compromised support, comfort, assistance, or encouragement that may be needed by the client to manage or master adaptive tasks related to his/her health challenge*

Defining Characteristics

Objective

- Significant person attempts assistive or supportive behaviors with less than satisfactory results
- Significant person displays protective behavior disproportionate (too little or too much) to client's abilities or need for autonomy
- Significant person withdraws or enters into limited or temporary personal communication with client at the time of need

Subjective

- Client expresses or confirms a concern or complaint about significant other's response to his/her health problem
- Significant person describes or confirms an inadequate understanding or knowledge base, which interferes with effective assistive or supportive behaviors
- Significant person describes preoccupation with personal reaction (e.g., fear, anticipatory grief, guilt, anxiety) to client's illness, disability, or other situational or developmental crisis

* *Formerly "Ineffective Family Coping: Compromised"*

Related Factors

C

Temporary preoccupation by a significant person who tries to manage emotional conflicts and personal suffering and is unable to perceive or act effectively in regard to client's needs

Temporary family disorganization and role changes

Prolonged disease or progression of disability that exhausts supportive capacity of significant people

Other situational or developmental crises or situations the significant person may be facing

Inadequate or incorrect information or understanding by a primary person

Little support provided by client, in turn, for primary person

C

DISABLED FAMILY COPING*
(1980, 1996)

Definition *Behavior of significant person (family member or other primary person) that disables his/her capacities and the client's capacities to effectively address tasks essential to either person's adaption to the health challenge*

Defining Characteristics

- Intolerance
- Agitation, depression, aggression, hostility
- Taking on illness signs of client
- Rejection
- Psychosomaticism
- Neglectful relationships with other family members
- Neglectful care of client in regard to basic human needs and/or illness treatment
- Distortion of reality regarding client's health problem, including extreme denial about its existence or severity
- Impaired restructuring of a meaningful life for self
- Impaired individualization, prolonged overconcern for client
- Desertion
- Decisions and actions by family that are detrimental to economic or social well-being
- Carrying on usual routines, disregarding client's needs
- Abandonment
- Client's development of helpless, inactive dependence
- Disregarding needs

* *Formerly "Ineffective Family Coping: Disabling"*

Related Factors

Significant person with chronically unexpressed feelings of quilt, anxiety, hostility, despair, etc.

Arbitrary handling of family's resistance to treatment, which tends to solidify defensiveness as it fails to deal adequately with underlying anxiety

Dissonant or discrepant coping styles for dealing with adaptive tasks by the significant person and client or among significant people

Highly ambivalent family relationships

C

READINESS FOR ENHANCED FAMILY COPING*
(1980)

Definition *Effective management of adaptive tasks by family member involved with the client's health challenge, who now exhibits desire and readiness for enhanced health and growth in regard to self and in relation to the client*

Defining Characteristics

- Individual expresses interest in making contact on a one-to-one basis or on a mutual-aid group basis with another person who has experienced a similar situation
- Family member attempts to describe growth impact of crisis on his/her own values, priorities, goal, or relationships

- Family member moves in direction of health-promoting and enriching life-style that supports and monitors maturational processes, audits and negotiates treatment programs, and chooses experiences that optimize wellness

Related Factors

Needs sufficiently gratified and adaptive tasks effectively addressed to enable goals of self-actualization to surface

---

* Formerly "Family Coping: Potential for Growth"

INEFFECTIVE DENIAL
(1988)

Definition *Conscious or unconscious attempt to disavow the knowledge or meaning of an event to reduce anxiety/fear, but leading to the detriment of health*

Defining Characteristics

- Delays seeking or refuses healthcare attention to the detriment of health
- Does not perceive personal relevance of symptoms or danger
- Displaces source of symptoms to other organs
- Displays inappropriate affect
- Does not admit fear of death or invalidism
- Makes dismissive gestures or comments when speaking of distressing events
- Minimizes symptoms
- Unable to admit impact of disease on life pattern
- Uses home remedies (self-treatment) to relieve symptoms
- Displaces fear of impact of the condition

Related Factors

To be developed

IMPAIRED DENTITION*
(1998)

Definition *Disruption in tooth development/eruption patterns or structural integrity of individual teeth*

Defining Characteristics

- Excessive plaque
- Crown or root caries
- Halitosis
- Tooth enamel discoloration
- Toothache
- Loose teeth
- Excessive calculus
- Incomplete eruption for age (may be primary or permanent teeth)
- Malocclusion or tooth misalignment
- Premature loss of primary teeth
- Worn down or abraded teeth
- Tooth fracture(s)
- Missing teeth or complete absence
- Erosion of enamel
- Asymmetrical facial expression

Related Factors

Ineffective oral hygiene, sensitivity to heat or cold
Barriers to self-care
Access or economic barriers to professional care
Nutritional deficits
Dietary habits
Genetic predisposition
Selected prescription medications
Premature loss of primary teeth

Excessive intake of fluorides
Chronic vomiting
Chronic use of tobacco, coffee or tea, red wine
Lack of knowledge regarding dental health
Excessive use of abrasive cleaning agents
Bruxism

* *Formerly "Altered Dentition"*

RISK FOR DELAYED DEVELOPMENT*
(1998)

D

Definition *At risk for delay of 25% or more in one or more of the areas of social or self-regulatory behavior, or in cognitive, language, gross or fine motor skills*

Risk Factors

Prenatal

Maternal age <15 or >35 years

Substance abuse

Infections

Genetic or endocrine disorders

Unplanned or unwanted pregnancy

Lack of, late, or poor prenatal care

Inadequate nutrition

Illiteracy

Poverty

Individual

Prematurity

Seizures

Congenital or genetic disorders

Positive drug screening test

Brain damage (e.g., hemorrhage in postnatal period, shaken baby, abuse, accident)

Vision impairment

Hearing impairment or frequent otitis media

Chronic illness

Technology-dependent

Failure to thrive, inadequate nutrition

Foster or adopted child

Lead poisoning

Chemotherapy

Radiation therapy

Natural disaster

Behavior disorders

Substance abuse

Environmental

Poverty

Violence

Caregiver

Abuse

Mental illness

Mental retardation or severe learning disability

* Formerly "Risk for Altered Development"

DIARRHEA
(1975, 1998)

D

Definition *Passage of loose, unformed stools*

Defining Characteristics
- At least 3 loose liquid stools per day
- Hyperactive bowel sounds
- Urgency
- Abdominal pain
- Cramping

Related Factors

Psychological

High stress levels and anxiety

Situational

Alcohol abuse
Toxins
Laxative abuse
Radiation
Tube feedings
Adverse effects of medications
Contaminants
Travel

Physiological

Inflammation
Malabsorption
Infectious processes
Irritation
Parasites

RISK FOR DISUSE SYNDROME
(1988)

Definition   *At risk for deterioration of body systems as the result of prescribed or unavoidable musculoskeletal inactivity*

Risk Factors
Severe pain
Mechanical
  immobilization
Altered level of
  consciousness
Prescribed immobilization
Paralysis

Note.   Complications from immobility can include pressure ulcer, constipation, stasis of pulmonary secretions, thrombosis, urinary tract infection and/or retention, decreased strength or endurance, orthostatic hypotension, decreased range of joint motion, disorientation, body-image disturbance, and powerlessness.

DEFICIENT DIVERSIONAL ACTIVITY*
(1980)

Definition *Decreased stimulation from (or interest or engagement in) recreational or leisure activities*

Defining Characteristics
- Usual hobbies cannot be undertaken in hospital
- Patient's statements regarding: boredom, wish there was something to do, to read, etc.

Related Factors
Environmental lack of diversional activity as in long-term hospitalization, frequent lengthy treatments

* Formerly " Diversional Activity Deficit"

DISTURBED ENERGY FIELD*
(1994)

E

Definition *Disruption of the flow of energy surrounding a person's being that results in disharmony of the body, mind, and/or spirit*

Defining Characteristics

- Movement (wave/spike/ tingling/dense/flowing)
- Sounds (tone/words)
- Temperature change (warmth/coolness)
- Visual changes (image/ color)
- Disruption of the field (vacant/hold/spike/ bulge)

Related Factors

To be developed

* *Formerly " Energy Field Disturbance"*

IMPAIRED **E**NVIRONMENTAL INTERPRETATION SYNDROME
(1994)

E

Definition *Consistent lack of orientation to person, place, time, or circumstances over more than 3 to 6 months necessitating a protective environment*

Defining Characteristics

- Consistent disorientation in known and unknown environments
- Chronic confusional states
- Loss of occupation or social functioning from memory decline
- Inability to follow simple directions, instructions
- Inability to concentrate
- Inability to reason
- Slow in responding to questions

Related Factors

Depression
Huntington's disease
Dementia (e.g.,
    Alzheimer's, multi-
    infarct, Pick's disease,
    AIDS, alcoholism,
    Parkinson's disease)

ADULT **F**AILURE TO THRIVE
(1998)

Definition   *Progressive functional deterioration of a physical and cognitive nature. The individual's ability to live with multisystem diseases, cope with ensuing problems, and manage his/her care are remarkably diminished.*

Defining Characteristics

- Anorexia: Does not eat meals when offered
- States does not have an appetite, not hungry, or "I don't want to eat"
- Inadequate nutritional intake: Eating less than body requirements
- Consumption of minimal to no food at most meals (i.e., consumes <75% of normal requirements)
- Weight loss (decreased from baseline weight)
  - 5% unintentional weight loss in 1 month
  - 10% unintentional weight loss in 6 months
- Physical decline (decline in bodily function): Evidence of fatigue, dehydration, incontinence of bowel and bladder
- Frequent exacerbations of chronic health problems (e.g., pneumonia, urinary tract infections)
- Cognitive decline (decline in mental processing) as evidenced by:
  - Problems with responding appropriately to environmental stimuli
  - Demonstrated difficulty in reasoning, decision making, judgment, memory and concentration
  - Decreased perception
- Decreased social skills/ social withdrawal: Noticeable decrease from usual past behavior in attempts to form or participate in cooperative

continued

Adult Failure to Thrive, *continued*

and interdependent relationships (e.g., decreased verbal communication with staff, family, friends)
- Decreased participation in activities of daily living that the older person once enjoyed
- Self-care deficit: No longer looks after or takes charge of physical cleanliness or appearance
- Difficulty performing simple self-care tasks
- Neglect of home environment and/or financial responsibilities

- Apathy as evidenced by lack of observable feeling or emotion in terms of normal activities of daily living and environment
- Altered mood state: Expresses feelings of sadness, being low in spirit
- Expresses loss of interest in pleasurable outlets such as food, sex, work, friends, family, hobbies, or entertainment
- Verbalizes desire for death

Related Factors

Depression
Apathy
Fatigue

RISK FOR FALLS
(2000)

Definition *Increased susceptibility to falling that may cause physical harm*

Risk Factors

Adults

History of falls
Wheelchair use
Age 65 or over
Female (if elderly)
Lives alone
Lower limb prosthesis
Use of assistive devices
(e.g., walker, cane)

Physiological

Presence of acute illness
Postoperative conditions
Visual difficulties
Hearing difficulties
Arthritis
Orthostatic hypotension
Sleeplessness
Faintness when turning
or extending neck
Anemias
Vascular disease
Neoplasms (i.e.,
fatigue/limited mobility)
Urgency and/or
incontinence
Diarrhea
Decreased lower
extremity strength
Postprandial blood sugar
changes

Foot problems
Impaired physical mobility
Impaired balance
Difficulty with gait
Proprioceptive deficits
(e.g., unilateral neglect)
Neuropathy

Cognitive

Diminished mental status
(e.g., confusion,
delirium, dementia,
impaired reality testing)

Medications

Antihypertensive agents
ACE inhibitors
Diuretics
Tricyclic antidepressants
Alcohol use
Antianxiety agents
Narcotics
Hypnotics or tranquilizers

Environment

Restraints
Weather conditions (e.g.,
wet floors/ice)
Throw/scatter rugs
Cluttered environment
Unfamiliar, dimly lit room
continued

Risk for Falls, *continued*

No antislip material in bath and/or shower

Children

<2 years of age
Male gender when <1 year of age
Lack of auto restraints

Lack of gate on stairs
Lack of window guard
Bed located near window
Unattended infant on bed/changing table/sofa
Lack of parental supervision

DYSFUNCTIONAL FAMILY PROCESSES: ALCOHOLISM*
(1994)

Definition *Psychosocial, spiritual, and physiological functions of the family unit are chronically disorganized, which leads to conflict, denial of problems, resistance to change, ineffective problem solving, and a series of self-perpetuating crises*

F

Defining Characteristics
Roles and Relationships
- Inconsistent parenting/ low perception of parental support
- Ineffective spouse communication/marital problems
- Intimacy dysfunction
- Deterioration in family relationships/disturbed family dynamics
- Altered role function/ disruption of family roles
- Closed communication systems
- Chronic family problems
- Family denial
- Lack of cohesiveness
- Neglected obligations
- Lack of skills necessary for relationships
- Reduced ability of family members to relate to each other for mutual growth and maturation
- Disrupted family rituals
- Family unable to meet security needs of its members
- Economic problems
- Family does not demonstrate respect for individuality and autonomy of its members
- Triangulating family relationships
- Pattern of rejection

Behavioral
- Refusal to get help/ inability to accept and receive help appropriately
- Inadequate understanding or knowledge of alcoholism
- Ineffective problem-solving skills
- Manipulation

continued

* *Formerly "Altered Family Processes: Alcoholism"*

Dysfunctional Family Processes:
Alcoholism, *continued*

- Rationalization/denial of problems
- Blaming, criticizing
- Inability to meet emotional needs of its members
- Alcohol abuse
- Broken promises
- Dependency
- Impaired communication
- Difficulty with intimate relationships
- Enabling to maintain alcoholic drinking pattern
- Inappropriate expression of anger
- Isolation
- Inability to meet spiritual needs of its members
- Inability to express or accept wide range of feelings
- Inability to deal constructively with traumatic experiences
- Inability to adapt to change
- Immaturity
- Harsh self-judgment
- Lying
- Lack of dealing with conflict
- Lack of reliability
- Nicotine addiction
- Orientation toward tension relief rather than achievement of goals
- Seeking approval and affirmation
- Difficulty having fun
- Agitation
- Chaos
- Contradictory, paradoxical communication
- Diminished physical contact
- Disturbances in academic performance in children
- Disturbances in concentration
- Escalating conflict
- Failure to accomplish current or past developmental tasks/difficulty with life cycle transitions
- Family special occasions are alcohol centered
- Controlling communication/power struggles
- Self-blaming
- Stress-related physical illnesses
- Substance abuse other than alcohol
- Unresolved grief
- Verbal abuse of spouse or parent

Feelings

- Insecurity
- Lingering resentment
- Mistrust
- Vulnerability
- Rejection
- Repressed emotions
- Responsibility for alcoholic's behavior
- Shame/embarrassment
- Unhappiness
- Powerlessness
- Anger/suppressed rage
- Anxiety, tension, or distress
- Emotional isolation/ loneliness
- Frustration
- Guilt
- Hopelessness
- Hurt
- Decreased self-esteem/ worthlessness
- Hostility
- Lack of identity
- Fear
- Loss
- Emotional control by others
- Misunderstood
- Moodiness
- Abandonment
- Being different from other people
- Being unloved
- Confused love and pity
- Confusion
- Failure
- Depression
- Dissatisfaction

Related Factors

Abuse of alcohol
Genetic predisposition
Lack of problem-solving skills
Inadequate coping skills

Family history of alcoholism, resistance to treatment
Biochemical influences
Addictive personality

INTERRUPTED FAMILY PROCESSES*
(1982, 1998)

Definition *Change in family relationships and/or functioning*

Defining Characteristics

- Changes in
  - Power alliances
  - Assigned tasks
  - Effectiveness in completing assigned tasks
  - Mutual support
  - Availability for affective responsiveness and intimacy
  - Patterns and rituals
  - Participation in problem solving
  - Participation in decision making
  - Communication patterns
  - Availability for emotional support
  - Satisfaction with family
  - Stress-reduction behaviors
  - Expressions of conflict with and/or isolation from community resources
  - Somatic complaints
  - Expressions of conflict within family

Related Factors

Power shift of family members
Family roles shift
Shift in health status of a family member
Developmental transition and/or crisis
Situation transition and/or crises
Informal or formal interaction with community
Modification in family social status
Modification in family finances

* Formerly "Altered Family Processes"

FATIGUE
(1988, 1998)

Definition *An overwhelming sustained sense of exhaustion and decreased capacity for physical and mental work at usual level*

Defining Characteristics

- Inability to restore energy even after sleep
- Lack of energy or inability to maintain usual level of physical activity
- Increase in rest requirements
- Tired
- Verbalization of an unremitting and overwhelming lack of energy
- Inability to maintain usual routines
- Lethargic or listless
- Increase in physical complaints
- Perceived need for additional energy to accomplish routine tasks
- Compromised concentration
- Disinterest in surroundings, introspection
- Decreased performance
- Compromised libido
- Drowsy
- Feelings of guilt for not keeping up with responsibilities

Related Factors

Psychological

Boring lifestyle
Stress
Anxiety
Depression

Environmental

Humidity
Lights
Noise
Temperature

Situational

Negative life events
Occupation

Physiological

Sleep deprivation
Pregnancy
Poor physical condition
Disease states
Increased physical exertion
Malnutrition
Anemia

FEAR
(1980, 1996, 2000)

Definition *Response to perceived threat that is consciously recognized as a danger*

Defining Characteristics

- Report of
  - Apprehension
  - Increased tension
  - Decreased self-assurance
  - Excitement
  - Being scared
  - Jitteriness
  - Dread
  - Alarm
  - Terror
  - Panic

Cognitive

- Identifies object of fear
- Stimulus believed to be a threat
- Diminished productivity, learning ability, problem-solving ability

Behaviors

- Increased alertness
- Avoidance or attack behaviors
- Impulsiveness
- Narrowed focus on "it" (i.e., the focus of the fear)

Physiological

- Increased pulse
- Anorexia
- Nausea
- Vomiting
- Diarrhea
- Muscle tightness
- Fatigue
- Increased respiratory rate and shortness of breath
- Pallor
- Increased perspiration
- Increased systolic blood pressure
- Pupil dilation
- Dry mouth

Related Factors

Natural/innate origin (e.g., sudden noise, height, pain, loss of physical support)

Learned response (e.g., conditioning, modeling from or identification with others)

Separation from support system in potentially stressful situation (e.g., hospitalization, hospital procedures)

Unfamiliarity with environmental experience(s)

Language barrier

Sensory impairment

Innate releasers (neurotransmitters)

Phobic stimulus

DEFICIENT FLUID VOLUME*
(1978, 1996)

Definition *Decreased intravascular, interstitial, and/or intracellular fluid. This refers to dehydration, water loss alone without change in sodium.*

F

Defining Characteristics

- Weakness
- Thirst
- Decreased skin/tongue turgor
- Dry skin/mucous membranes
- Increased pulse rate, decreased blood pressure, decreased pulse volume/pressure
- Decreased venous filling
- Change in mental state
- Decreased urine output
- Increased urine concentration
- Increased body temperature
- Elevated hematocrit
- Sudden weight loss (except in third spacing)

Related Factors

Active fluid volume loss
Failure of regulatory
  mechanisms

* Formerly "Fluid Volume Deficit"

EXCESS FLUID VOLUME*
(1982, 1996)

Definition *Increased isotonic fluid retention*

Defining Characteristics

- Weight gain over short period of time
- Intake exceeds output
- Blood pressure changes, pulmonary artery pressure changes, increased central venous pressure
- Edema, may progress to anascara
- Jugular vein distention
- Changes in respiratory pattern, dyspnea or shortness of breath, orthopnea, abnormal breath sounds (rales or crackles), pulmonary congestion, pleural effusion
- Decreased hemoglobin and hematocrit, altered electrolytes, specific gravity changes
- S3 heart sound
- Positive hepatojugular reflex
- Oliguria, azotemia
- Change in mental status, restlessness, anxiety

Related Factors

Compromised regulatory mechanism
Excess fluid intake
Excess sodium intake

* *Formerly "Fluid Volume Excess"*

RISK FOR DEFICIENT FLUID VOLUME*
(1978)

Definition *At risk for experiencing vascular, cellular, or intracellular dehydration*

Risk Factors

Factors influencing fluids needs (e.g., hypermetabolic state)

Medication (e.g., diuretics)

Loss of fluid through abnormal routes (e.g., indwelling tubes)

Knowledge deficiency related to fluid volume

Extremes of age

Deviations affecting access, intake, or absorption of fluids (e.g., physical immobility)

Extremes of weight

Excessive losses through normal routes (e.g., diarrhea)

* Formerly "Risk for Fluid Volume Deficit"

RISK FOR IMBALANCED FLUID VOLUME*
(1998)

Definition   At risk for a decrease, increase, or rapid shift from one to the other of intravascular, interstitial, and/or intracellular fluid. This refers to body fluid loss, gain, or both.

Risk Factors

Scheduled for major
   invasive procedures
Other risk factors to be
   determined

* Formerly "Risk for Fluid Volume Imbalance"

IMPAIRED GAS EXCHANGE
(1980, 1996, 1998)

Definition *Excess or deficit in oxygenation and/or carbon dioxide elimination at the alveolar-capillary membrane*

Defining Characteristics

- Visual disturbances
- Decreased carbon dioxide
- Tachycardia
- Hypercapnia
- Restlessness
- Somnolence
- Irritability
- Hypoxia
- Confusion
- Dyspnea
- Abnormal arterial blood gases
- Cyanosis (in neonates only)
- Abnormal skin color (pale, dusky)
- Hypoxemia
- Hypercarbia
- Headache upon awakening
- Abnormal rate, rhythm, depth of breathing
- Diaphoresis
- Abnormal arterial pH
- Nasal flaring

Related Factors

Ventilation perfusion imbalance
Alveolar-capillary membrane changes

ANTICIPATORY GRIEVING
(1980, 1996)

Definition *Intellectual and emotional responses and behaviors by which individuals, families, communities work through the process of modifying self-concept based on the perception of potential loss*

Defining Characteristics

- Potential loss of significant object (e.g., people, possessions, job, status, home, ideals, parts and processes of the body)
- Expression of distress at potential loss
- Sorrow
- Guilt
- Denial of potential loss
- Anger
- Altered communication patterns
- Denial of the significance of the loss
- Bargaining
- Alteration in eating habits, sleep patterns, dream patterns, activity level, libido
- Difficulty taking on new or different roles
- Resolution of grief prior to the reality of loss

Related Factors

To be developed

DYSFUNCTIONAL GRIEVING
(1980, 1996)

Definition *Extended, unsuccessful use of intellectual and emotional responses by which individuals, families, communities attempt to work through the process of modifying self-concept based upon the perception of loss*

Defining Characteristics

- Repetitive use of ineffectual behaviors associated with attempts to reinvest in relationships
- Reliving of past experiences with little or no reduction (diminishment) of intensity of the grief
- Prolonged interference with life functioning
- Onset or exacerbation of somatic or psychosomatic responses
- Verbal expression of distress at loss
- Denial of loss
- Expression of guilt
- Expression of unresolved issues
- Anger
- Sadness
- Crying
- Difficulty in expressing loss
- Alterations in eating habits, sleep patterns, dream patterns, activity level, libido, concentration and/or pursuit of tasks
- Idealization of lost object (e.g., people, possessions, job, status, home, ideals, parts and processes of the body)
- Interference with life functioning
- Developmental regression
- Labile affect

Related Factors

Actual or perceived object loss (e.g., people, possessions, job, status, home, ideals, parts and processes of the body)

DELAYED GROWTH AND DEVELOPMENT*
(1986)

Definition *Deviations from age-group norms*

Defining Characteristics

- Altered physical growth
- Delay or difficulty in performing skills (motor, social, expressive) typical of age group
- Inability to perform self-care or self-control activities appropriate for age
- Flat affect
- Listlessness, decreased response time

G

Related Factors

Prescribed dependence
Indifference
Separation from significant others
Environmental and stimulation deficiencies

Effects of physical disability
Inadequate caretaking
Inconsistent responsiveness
Multiple caretakers

---

* *Formerly "Altered Growth and Development"*

RISK FOR DISPROPORTIONATE Growth*
(1998)

Definition *At risk for growth above the 97th percentile or below the 3rd percentile for age, crossing two percentile channels; disproportionate growth*

Risk Factors

Prenatal

Congenital/genetic
disorders
Maternal nutrition
Multiple gestation
Teratogen exposure
Substance use/abuse
Maternal infection

Individual

Infection
Prematurity
Malnutrition
Organic and inorganic
factors
Caregiver and/or
individual maladaptive
feeding behaviors
Anorexia
Insatiable appetite
Chronic illness
Substance abuse

Environmental

Deprivation
Teratogen
Lead poisoning
Poverty
Violence
Natural disasters

Caregiver

Abuse
Mental illness, mental
retardation, severe
learning disability

---

* Formerly "Risk for Altered Growth"

INEFFECTIVE HEALTH MAINTENANCE*
(1982)

Definition *Inability to identify, manage and/or seek out help to maintain health*

Defining Characteristics

- Demonstrated lack of knowledge regarding basic health practices
- Demonstrated lack of adaptive behaviors to internal/external environmental changes
- Reported or observed inability to take responsibility for meeting basic health practices in any or all functional pattern areas
- History of lack of health-seeking behavior
- Expressed interest in improving health behaviors
- Reported or observed lack of equipment, financial and/or other resources
- Reported or observed impairment of personal support systems

Related Factors

Ineffective family coping
Perceptual/cognitive impairment (complete/partial lack of gross and/or fine motor skills)
Lack of, or significant alteration in, communication skills (written, verbal, and/or gestural)

Unachieved developmental tasks
Lack of material resources
Dysfunctional grieving
Disabling spiritual distress
Lack of ability to make deliberate and thoughtful judgments
Ineffective individual coping

* *Formerly "Altered Health Maintenance"*

HEALTH-SEEKING BEHAVIORS (Specify)
(1988)

Definition   *Active seeking (by a person in stable health) of ways to alter personal health habits and/or the environment in order to move toward a higher level of health*

Defining Characteristics

- Expressed or observed desire to seek a higher level of wellness
- Demonstrated or observed lack of knowledge about health-promotion behaviors
- Stated or observed unfamiliarity with wellness community resources
- Expression of concern about current environmental conditions on health status
- Expressed or observed desire for increased control of health practice

Related Factors

To be developed

Note.   Stable health is defined as achievement of age-appropriate illness-prevention measures; client reports good or excellent health, and signs and symptoms of disease, if present, are controlled.

IMPAIRED HOME MAINTENANCE*
(1980)

Definition *Inability to independently maintain a safe growth-promoting immediate environment*

Defining Characteristics

Subjective

- Household members express difficulty in maintaining their home in a comfortable fashion
- Household members describe outstanding debts or financial crises
- Household members request assistance with home maintenance

Objective

- Disorderly surroundings
- Unwashed or unavailable cooking equipment, clothes, or linen

- Accumulation of dirt, food wastes, or hygienic wastes
- Offensive odors
- Inappropriate household temperature
- Overtaxed family members (e.g., exhausted, anxious)
- Lack of necessary equipment or aids
- Presence of vermin or rodents
- Repeated hygienic disorders, infestations, or infections

Related Factors

Individual/family member disease or injury
Unfamiliarity with neighborhood resources
Lack of role modeling
Lack of knowledge
Insufficient family organization or planning

Inadequate support systems
Impaired cognitive or emotional functioning
Insufficient finances

---

* *Formerly "Impaired Home Maintenance Management"*

HOPELESSNESS
(1986)

Definition   *Subjective state in which an individual sees limited or no alternatives or personal choices available and is unable to mobilize energy on own behalf*

Defining Characteristics

- Passivity, decreased verbalization
- Decreased affect
- Verbal cues (e.g., despondent content, "I can't," sighing)
- Closing eyes
- Decreased appetite
- Decreased response to stimuli
- Increased/decreased sleep
- Lack of initiative
- Lack of involvement in care/passively allowing care
- Shrugging in response to speaker
- Turning away from speaker

Related Factors

Abandonment

Prolonged activity restriction creating isolation

Lost belief in transcendent values/God

Long-term stress

Failing or deteriorating physiological condition

HYPERTHERMIA
(1986)

Definition *Body temperature elevated above normal range*

Defining Characteristics

- Increase in body temperature above normal range
- Seizures or convulsions
- Flushed skin
- Increased respiratory rate
- Tachycardia
- Warm to touch

Related Factors

Illness or trauma
Increased metabolic rate
Vigorous activity
Medications or anesthesia
Inability or decreased ability to perspire

Exposure to hot environment
Dehydration
Inappropriate clothing

Hypothermia
(1986, 1988)

Definition *Body temperature below normal range*

Defining Characteristics

- Reduction in body temperature below normal range
- Pallor
- Shivering
- Cool skin
- Cyanotic nail beds
- Hypertension
- Piloerection
- Slow capillary refill
- Tachycardia

Related Factors

Exposure to cool or cold environment
Medications causing vasodilation
Malnutrition
Inadequate clothing
Illness or trauma
Evaporation from skin in cool environment
Decreased metabolic rate
Damage to hypothalamus
Consumption of alcohol
Aging
Inability or decreased ability to shiver
Inactivity

DISTURBED PERSONAL IDENTITY*
(1978)

Definition *Inability to distinguish between self and nonself*

Defining Characteristics
• To be developed

Related Factors
To be developed

---

* *Formerly "Personal Identity Disturbance"*

FUNCTIONAL URINARY INCONTINENCE
(1986, 1998)

Definition *Inability of usually continent person to reach toilet in time to avoid unintentional loss of urine*

Defining Characteristics

- Amount of time required to reach toilet exceeds length of time between sensing the urge to void and uncontrolled voiding
- Loss of urine before reaching toilet
- May only be incontinent in early morning
- Senses need to void
- Able to completely empty bladder

Related Factors

Psychological factors
Impaired vision
Impaired cognition
Neuromuscular limitations

Altered environmental factors
Weakened supporting pelvic structures

REFLEX URINARY INCONTINENCE
(1986, 1998)

Definition *Involuntary loss of urine at somewhat predictable intervals when a specific bladder volume is reached*

Defining Characteristics

- No sensation of urge to void
- Complete emptying with lesion above pontine micturition center
- Incomplete emptying with lesion above sacral micturition center
- No sensation of bladder fullness
- Sensations associated with full bladder such as sweating, restlessness, and abdominal discomfort
- Inability to voluntarily inhibit or initiate voiding
- No sensation of voiding
- Predictable pattern of voiding
- Sensation of urgency without voluntary inhibition of bladder contraction

Related Factors

Tissue damage from radiation cystitis, inflammatory bladder conditions, or radical pelvic surgery

Neurological impairment above level of sacral or pontine micturition center

STRESS URINARY INCONTINENCE*
(1986)

Definition *Loss of less than 50 ml of urine occurring with increased abdominal pressure*

Defining Characteristics
- Reported or observed dribbling with increased abdominal pressure
- Urinary frequency (more often than every 2 hours)
- Urinary urgency

Related Factors
Weak pelvic muscles and structural supports

Degenerative changes in pelvic muscles and structural supports associated with increased age

High intra-abdominal pressure (e.g., obesity, gravid uterus)

Overdistention between voidings

Incompetent bladder outlet

TOTAL URINARY INCONTINENCE*
(1986)

Definition   *Continuous and unpredictable loss of urine*

Defining Characteristics

- Constant flow of urine at unpredictable times without uninhibited bladder contractions/spasm or distention
- Nocturia
- Unsuccessful incontinence refractory treatments
- Unawareness of incontinence
- Lack of perineal or bladder filling awareness

Related Factors

Neuropathy preventing transmission of reflex indicating bladder fullness

Trauma or disease affecting spinal cord nerves

Anatomic (fistula)

Independent contraction of detrusor reflex due to surgery

Neurological dysfunction causing triggering of micturition at unpredictable times

---

* Formerly "Total Incontinence"

URGE URINARY INCONTINENCE*
(1986)

Definition *Involuntary passage of urine occurring soon after a strong sense of urgency to void*

Defining Characteristics

- Urinary urgency
- Bladder contracture/spasm
- Frequency (voiding more often than every 2 hours)
- Voiding in large amounts (>550 cc)
- Voiding in small amounts (<100 cc)
- Nocturia (more than 2 times a night)
- Inability to reach toilet in time

Related Factors

Alcohol
Caffeine
Decreased bladder capacity (e.g., history of PID, abdominal surgeries, indwelling urinary catheter)
Increased fluids

Increased urine concentration
Irritation of bladder stretch receptors causing spasm (e.g., bladder infection)
Overdistention of bladder

---

* *Formerly "Urge Incontinence"*

RISK FOR URGE URINARY INCONTINENCE*
(1998)

Definition *At risk for involuntary loss of urine associated with a sudden, strong sensation or urinary urgency*

Risk Factors

Effects of medications, caffeine, alcohol

Detrusor hyperreflexia from cystitis, urethritis, tumors, renal calculi, central nervous system disorders above pontine micturition center

Detrusor muscle instability with impaired contractility

Involuntary sphincter relaxation

Ineffective toileting habits

Small bladder capacity

* *Formerly "Risk for Urinary Urge Incontinence"*

DISORGANIZED INFANT BEHAVIOR
(1994, 1998)

Definition *Disintegrated physiological and neurobehavioral responses to the environment*

Defining Characteristics

Regulatory Problems
- Inability to inhibit startle
- Irritability

State-Organization System
- Active-awake (fussy, worried gaze)
- Diffuse/unclear sleep, state-oscillation
- Quiet-awake (staring, gaze aversion)
- Irritable or panicky crying

Attention-Interaction System
- Abnormal response to sensory stimuli (e.g., difficult to soothe, inability to sustain alert status)

Motor System
- Increased, decreased, or limp tone
- Finger splay, fisting or hands to face
- Hyperextension of arms and legs

- Tremors, startles, twitches
- Jittery, jerky, uncoordinated movement
- Altered primitive reflexes

Physiological
- Bradycardia, tachycardia, or arrhythmias
- Pale, cyanotic, mottled, or flushed color
- "Time-out signals" (e.g., gaze, grasp, hiccough, cough, sneeze, sigh, slack jaw, open mouth, tongue thrust)
- Oximeter reading: Desaturation
- Feeding intolerances (aspiration or emesis)

Related Factors

Prenatal

Congenital or genetic
  disorders
Teratogenic exposure

Postnatal

Malnutrition
Oral/motor problems
Pain
Feeding intolerance
Invasive/painful
  procedures
Prematurity

Individual

Illness
Immature neurological
  system
Gestational age
Postconceptual age

Environmental

Physical environment
  inappropriateness
Sensory inappropriateness
Sensory overstimulation
Sensory deprivation

Caregiver

Cue misreading
Cue knowledge deficit
Environmental stimula-
  tion contribution

RISK FOR DISORGANIZED INFANT BEHAVIOR
(1994)

Definition *Risk for alteration in integrating and modulation of the physiological and behavioral systems of functioning (i.e., autonomic, motor, state, organizational, self-regulatory, and attentional-interactional systems)*

Risk Factors

Pain
Invasive/painful
  procedures
Lack of containment/
  boundaries
Oral/motor problems
Prematurity
Environmental
  overstimulation

READINESS FOR ENHANCED ORGANIZED INFANT BEHAVIOR*
(1994)

Definition *A pattern of modulation of the physiologic and behavioral systems of functioning (i.e., autonomic, motor, state-organizational, self-regulators, and attentional-interactional systems) in an infant that is satisfactory but that can be improved resulting in higher levels of integration in response to environmental stimuli*

Defining Characteristics

- Definite sleep-wake states
- Use of some self-regulatory behaviors
- Response to visual/auditory stimuli
- Stable physiologic measures

Related Factors

Pain
Prematurity

---

* *Formerly "Potential for Enhanced Organized Infant Behavior"*

INEFFECTIVE INFANT FEEDING PATTERN
(1992)

Definition *Impaired ability to suck or coordingate the suck-swallow response*

Defining Characteristics
- Inability to coordinate sucking, swallowing, and breathing
- Inability to initiate or sustain an effective suck

Related Factors
Prolonged NPO
Anatomic abnormality
Neurological impairment/
   delay
Oral hypersensitivity
Prematurity

RISK FOR INFECTION
(1986)

Definition *At increased risk for being invaded by pathogenic organisms*

Risk Factors

Invasive procedures
Insufficient knowledge to avoid exposure to pathogens
Trauma
Tissue destruction and increased environmental exposure
Rupture of amniotic membranes
Pharmaceutical agents (e.g., immunosuppressants)
Malnutrition
Increased environmental exposure to pathogens
Immunosuppression
Inadequate acquired immunity
Inadequate secondary defenses (decreased hemoglobin, leukopenia, suppressed inflammatory response)
Inadequate primary defenses (broken skin, traumatized tissue, decrease in ciliary action, stasis of body fluids, change in pH secretions, altered peristalsis)
Chronic disease

RISK FOR INJURY
(1978)

Definition *At risk of injury as a result of environmental conditions interacting with the individual's adaptive and defensive resources*

Risk Factors

External

Mode of transport or transportation

People or provider (e.g., nosocomial agents; staffing patterns; cognitive, affective, psychomotor factors)

Physical (e.g., design, structure, and arrangement of community, building, and/or equipment)

Nutrients (e.g., vitamins, food types)

Biological (e.g., immunization level of community, microorganism)

Chemical (e.g., pollutants, poisons, drugs, pharmaceutical agents, alcohol, caffeine, nicotine, preservatives, cosmetics, dyes)

Internal

Psychological (affective orientation)

Malnutrition

Abnormal blood profile (e.g., leukocytosis/leukopenia, altered clotting factors, thrombocytopenia, sickle cell, thalassemia, decreased hemoglobin)

Immune-autoimmune dysfunction

Biochemical, regulatory function (e.g., sensory dysfunction)

Integrative dysfunction

Effector dysfunction

Tissue hypoxia

Developmental age (physiological, psychosocial)

Physical (e.g., broken skin, altered mobility)

RISK FOR PERIOPERATIVE-POSITIONING INJURY
(1994)

Definition   *At risk for injury as a result of the environmental conditions found in the perioperative setting*

Risk Factors

Disorientation
Edema
Emaciation
Immobilization
Muscle weakness
Obesity
Sensory/perceptual
  disturbances due to
  anesthesia

DECREASED INTRACRANIAL ADAPTIVE CAPACITY*
(1994)

Definition *Intracranial fluid dynamic mechanisms that normally compensate for increases in intracranial volumes are compromised, resulting in repeated disproportionate increases in intracranial pressure (ICP) in response to a variety of noxious and nonnoxious stimuli*

Defining Characteristics

- Repeated increases of >10 mm Hg for more than 5 minutes following any of a variety of external stimuli
- Baseline ICP ≥10 mm Hg
- Disproportionate increase in ICP following single environmental or nursing maneuver stimulus
- Elevated P_2 ICP wave form
- Volume pressure response test variation (volume-pressure ratio 2, pressure-volume index <10)
- Wide amplitude ICP wave form

Related Factors

Decreased cerebral perfusion ≤50–60 mm Hg

Sustained increase in ICP = 10–15 mm Hg

Systemic hypotension with intracranial hypertension

Brain injuries

---

* Formerly "Decreased Adaptive Capacity: Intracranial"

DEFICIENT Knowledge (Specify)*
(1980)

Definition *Absence or deficiency of cognitive information related to a specific topic*

Defining Characteristics

- Verbalization of the problem
- Inaccurate follow-through of instruction
- Inaccurate performance of test

- Inappropriate or exaggerated behaviors (e.g., hysterical, hostile, agitated, apathetic)

Related Factors

Lack of exposure
Lack of recall
Information misinterpretation

Cognitive limitation
Lack of interest in learning
Unfamiliarity with information resources

* Formerly "Knowledge Deficit"

RISK FOR LONELINESS
(1994)

Definition   *At risk for experiencing vague dysphoria*

Risk Factors
Affectional deprivation
Social isolation
Cathectic deprivation
Physical isolation

IMPAIRED MEMORY
(1994)

Definition *Inability to remember or recall bits of information or behavioral skills.** *

Defining Characteristics

- Inability to recall factual information
- Inability to recall recent or past events
- Inability to learn or retain new skills or information
- Inability to determine if a behavior was performed

- Observed or reported experiences of forgetting
- Inability to perform a previously learned skill
- Forgets to perform a behavior at a scheduled time

Related Factors

Fluid and electrolyte imbalance
Neurological disturbances
Excessive environmental disturbances
Anemia
Acute or chronic hypoxia
Decreased cardiac output

M

* *Impaired memory may be attributed to pathophysiological or situational causes that are either temporary or permanent.*

IMPAIRED BED MOBILITY
(1998)

Definition *Limitation of independent movement from one bed position to another*

Defining Characteristics

- Impaired ability to
  - Turn side to side
  - Move from supine to sitting or sitting to supine
  - "Scoot" or reposition self in bed
  - Move from supine to prone or prone to supine
  - Move from supine to long sitting or long sitting to supine

M

IMPAIRED PHYSICAL MOBILITY
(1973, 1998)

Definition *Limitation in independent, purposeful physical movement of the body or of one or more extremities*

Defining Characteristics

- Postural instability during performance of routine activities of daily living
- Limited ability to perform gross motor skills
- Limited ability to perform fine motor skills
- Uncoordinated or jerky movements
- Limited range of motion
- Difficulty turning
- Gait changes (e.g., decreased walking speed, difficulty initiating gait, small steps, shuffles feet, exaggerated lateral postural sway)
- Decreased reaction time
- Movement-induced shortness of breath
- Engages in substitutions for movement (e.g., increased attention to other's activity, controlling behavior, focus on preillness disability/ activity)
- Slowed movement
- Movement-induced tremor

M

Related Factors

Medications
Prescribed movement restrictions
Discomfort, pain
Lack of knowledge regarding value of physical activity
Body mass index above 75th age-appropriate percentile

Sensoriperceptual impairments
Musculoskeletal, neuro-muscular impairment
Intolerance to activity/ decreased strength and endurance
Depressive mood state or anxiety

continued

Impaired Physical Mobility, *continued*

Cognitive impairment
Decreased muscle strength, control and/or mass
Reluctance to initiate movement
Sedentary lifestyle, disuse, deconditioning
Selective or generalized malnutrition
Loss of integrity of bone structures

Developmental delay
Joint stiffness or contractures
Limited cardiovascular endurance
Altered cellular metabolism
Lack of physical or social environmental supports
Cultural beliefs regarding age appropriate activity

Note. Suggested Functional Level Classification:
  0 = Completely independent
  1 = Requires use of equipment or device
  2 = Requires help from another person, for assistance, supervision, or teaching
  3 = Requires help from another person and equipment or device
  4 = Dependent, does not participate in activity

IMPAIRED WHEELCHAIR Mobility
(1998)

Definition   *Limitation of independent operation of wheelchair within environment*

Defining Characteristics

• Impaired ability to operate manual or power wheelchair on even or uneven surface
• Impaired ability to operate manual or power wheelchair on an incline or decline
• Impaired ability to operate wheelchair on curbs

Note. Specify level of independence.

Nausea
(1998)

Definition *Unpleasant, wavelike sensation in the back of the throat, epigastrium, or throughout the abdomen that may or may not lead to vomiting*

Defining Characteristics

- Reports of "nausea" or "sick to stomach"
- Usually precedes vomiting, but may be experienced after vomiting or when vomiting does not occur

- Accompanied by pallor, cold and clammy skin, increased salivation, tachycardia, gastric stasis, diarrhea
- Accompanied by swallowing movements affected by skeletal muscles

Related Factors

Chemotherapy
Postsurgical anesthesia
Irritation to the gastrointestinal system
Stimulation of neuropharmacologic mechanisms

UNILATERAL NEGLECT
(1986)

Definition *Lack of awareness and attention to one side of the body*

Defining Characteristics

- Consistent inattention to stimuli on an affected side
- Does not look toward affected side
- Leaves food on plate on the affected side
- Inadequate self-care
- Inadequate positioning and/or safety precautions in regard to the affected side

Related Factors

Effects of disturbed perceptual abilities (e.g., hemianopsia)
Neurologic illness or trauma
One-sided blindness

N

NONCOMPLIANCE
(1973, 1996, 1998)

Definition *Behavior of person and/or caregiver that fails to coincide with a health-promoting or therapeutic plan agreed on by the person (and/or family and/or community) and health-care professional. In the presence of an agreed-on, health-promoting or therapeutic plan, person's or caregiver's behavior is fully or partially nonadherent and may lead to clinically ineffective or partially ineffective outcomes.*

Defining Characteristics

- Behavior indicative of failure to adhere (by direct observation or by statements of patient or significant others)
- Evidence of development of complications
- Evidence of exacerbation of symptoms
- Failure to keep appointments
- Failure to progress
- Objective tests (e.g., physiological measures, detection of physiologic markers)

Related Factors

Healthcare Plan

Duration
Significant others
Cost
Intensity
Complexity

Individual Factors

Personal and developmental abilities
Health beliefs, cultural influences, spiritual values
Individual's value system
Knowledge and skill relevant to the regimen behavior
Motivational forces

Health System

Satisfaction with care
Credibility of provider
Access and convenience of care
Financial flexibility of plan
Client-provider relationships

Provider reimbursement of teaching and follow-up

Provider continuity and regular follow-up

Individual health coverage

Communication and teaching skills of the provider

Network

Involvement of members in health plan

Social value regarding plan

Perceived beliefs of significant others

N

IMBALANCED NUTRITION: LESS THAN BODY REQUIREMENTS*
(1975)

Definition *Intake of nutrients insufficient to meet metabolic needs*

Defining Characteristics

- Body weight 20% or more under ideal
- Reported food intake less than RDA (recommended daily allowance)
- Pale conjunctival and mucous membranes
- Weakness of muscles required for swallowing or mastication
- Sore, inflamed buccal cavity
- Satiety immediately after ingesting food
- Reported or evidence of lack of food
- Reported altered taste sensation
- Perceived inability to ingest food
- Misconceptions
- Loss of weight with adequate food intake
- Aversion to eating
- Abdominal cramping
- Poor muscle tone
- Abdominal pain with or without pathology
- Lack of interest in food
- Capillary fragility
- Diarrhea and/or steatorrhea
- Excessive loss of hair
- Hyperactive bowel sounds
- Lack of information, misinformation

Related Factors

Inability to ingest or digest food or absorb nutrients due to biological, psychological, or economic factors

* Formerly "Altered Nutrition: Less Than Body Requirements"

N

IMBALANCED NUTRITION: MORE THAN BODY REQUIREMENTS*
(1975)

Definition *Intake of nutrients that exceeds metabolic needs*

Defining Characteristics

- Triceps skin fold >25 mm in women, >15 mm in men
- Weight 20% over ideal for height and frame
- Eating in response to external cues (e.g., time of day, social situation)
- Eating in response to internal cues other than hunger (e.g., anxiety)
- Reported or observed dysfunctional eating pattern (e.g., pairing food with other activities)
- Sedentary activity level
- Concentrating food intake at the end of the day

Related Factors

Excessive intake in relation to metabolic need

N

---

* *Formerly "Altered Nutrition: More Than Body Requirements"*

RISK FOR IMBALANCED NUTRITION: MORE THAN BODY REQUIREMENTS*
(1980)

Definition *At risk for an intake of nutrients that exceeds metabolic needs*

Risk Factors

Reported use of solid food as major food source before 5 months of age

Concentrating food intake at end of day

Reported or observed obesity in one or both parents

Reported or observed higher baseline weight at beginning of each pregnancy

Rapid transition across growth percentiles in infants or children

Pairing food with other activities

Observed use of food as reward or comfort measure

Eating in response to internal cues other than hunger (e.g., anxiety)

Eating in response to external cues (e.g., time of day, social situation)

Dysfunctional eating patterns

N

---

* *Formerly "Altered Nutrition: Risk For More Than Body Requirements"*

O

IMPAIRED ORAL MUCOUS MEMBRANE*
(1982, 1998)

Definition   *Disruption of the lips and soft tissue of the oral cavity*

Defining Characteristics

- Purulent drainage or exudates
- Gingival recession, pockets deeper than 4 mm
- Enlarged tonsils beyond what is developmentally appropriate
- Smooth atrophic, sensitive tongue
- Geographic tongue
- Mucosal denudation
- Presence of pathogens
- Difficult speech
- Self-report of bad taste
- Gingival or mucosal pallor
- Oral pain/discomfort
- Xerostomia (dry mouth)
- Vesicles, nodules, or papules
- White patches/plaques, spongy patches, or white curdlike exudate
- Oral lesions or ulcers
- Halitosis
- Edema
- Hyperemia
- Desquamation
- Coated tongue
- Stomatitis
- Self-report of difficulty eating or swallowing
- Self-report of diminished or absent taste
- Bleeding
- Macroplasia
- Gingival hyperplasia
- Fissures, cheilitis
- Red or bluish masses (e.g., hemangiomas)

continued

O

---

* *Formerly "Altered Oral Mucous Membrane"*

Impaired Oral Mucous Membrane, *continued*

Related Factors

Chemotherapy
Chemical irritants (e.g., alcohol, tobacco, acidic foods, drugs, regular use of inhalers or other noxious agents)
Depression
Immunosuppression
Aging-related loss of connective, adipose, or bone tissue
Barriers to professional care
Cleft lip or palate
Medication side effects
Lack of or decreased salivation
Trauma
Pathological conditions: Oral cavity (radiation to head or neck)
NPO for more than 24 hours

Mouth breathing
Malnutrition or vitamin deficiency
Dehydration
Infection
Ineffective oral hygiene
Mechanical (e.g., ill-fitting dentures, braces, tubes [endotracheal/ nasogastric], surgery in oral cavity)
Decreased platelets
Immunocompromised
Radiation therapy
Barriers to oral self-care
Diminished hormone levels (women)
Stress
Loss of supportive structures

ACUTE PAIN*
(1996)

Definition *Unpleasant sensory and emotional experience arising from actual or potential tissue damage or described in terms of such damage (International Association for the Study of Pain); sudden or slow onset of any intensity from mild to severe with an anticipated or predictable end and a duration of less than 6 months*

Defining Characteristics

- Verbal or coded report
- Observed evidence
- Antalgic positioning to avoid pain
- Protective gestures
- Guarding behavior
- Facial mask
- Sleep disturbance (eyes lack luster, beaten look, fixed or scattered movement, grimace)
- Self-focus
- Narrowed focus (altered time perception, impaired thought processes, reduced interaction with people and environment)
- Distraction behavior (e.g., pacing, seeking out other people and/or activities, repetitive activities)
- Autonomic responses (e.g., diaphoresis; changes in blood pressure, respiration, pulse; pupillary dilation)
- Autonomic change in muscle tone (may span from listless to rigid)
- Expressive behavior (e.g., restlessness, moaning, crying, vigilance, irritability, sighing)
- Changes in appetite and eating

Related Factors

Injury agents (biological, chemical, physical, psychological)

* Formerly "Pain"

CHRONIC PAIN
(1986, 1996)

Definition *Unpleasant sensory and emotional experience arising from actual or potential tissue damage or described in terms of such damage (International Association for the Study of Pain); sudden or slow onset of any intensity from mild to severe, constant or recurring without an anticipated or predictable end and a duration of greater than 6 months*

Defining Characteristics

- Weight changes
- Verbal or coded report or observed evidence of protective behavior, guarding behavior, facial mask, irritability, self-focusing, restlessness, depression
- Atrophy of involved muscle group
- Changes in sleep pattern
- Fatigue
- Fear of reinjury
- Reduced interaction with people
- Altered ability to continue previous activities
- Sympathetic mediated responses (e.g., temperature, cold, changes of body position, hypersensitivity)
- Anorexia

Related Factors

Chronic physical/ psychosocial disability

IMPAIRED PARENTING*
(1978, 1998)

Definition *Inability of the primary caretaker to create, maintain, or regain an environment that promotes the optimum growth and development of the child*

Defining Characteristics

Infant or Child

- Poor academic performance
- Frequent illness
- Runaway
- Incidence of physical and psychological trauma or abuse
- Frequent accidents
- Lack of attachment
- Failure to thrive
- Behavioral disorders
- Poor social competence
- Lack of separation anxiety
- Poor cognitive development

Parental

- Inappropriate child care arrangements
- Rejection or hostility to child
- Statements of inability to meet child's needs
- Inflexibility in meeting needs of child or situation

- Poor or inappropriate caretaking skills
- Frequently punitive
- Inconsistent care
- Child abuse
- Inadequate child health maintenance
- Unsafe home environment
- Verbalization of inability to control child
- Negative statements about child
- Verbalization of role inadequacy or frustration
- Inappropriate visual, tactile, auditory stimulation
- Abandonment
- Insecure (or lack of) attachment to infant
- Inconsistent behavior management
- Child neglect
- Little cuddling
- Maternal-child interaction deficit
- Poor parent-child interaction

continued

* *Formerly "Altered Parenting"*

Impaired Parenting, *continued*

Related Factors

Social

Lack of access to resources

Social isolation

Lack of resources

Poor home environment

Lack of family cohesiveness

Inadequate child care arrangements

Lack of transportation

Unemployment or job problems

Role strain or overload

Marital conflict, declining satisfaction

Lack of value of parenthood

Change in family unit

Low socioeconomic class

Unplanned or unwanted pregnancy

Presence of stress (e.g., financial, legal, recent crisis, cultural move)

Lack of, or poor, parental role model

Single parent

Lack of social support networks

Father of child not involved

History of being abusive

History of being abused

Financial difficulties

Maladaptive coping strategies

Poverty

Poor problem-solving skills

Inability to put child's needs before own

Low self-esteem

Relocations

Legal difficulties

Knowledge

Lack of knowledge about child health maintenance

Lack of knowledge about parenting skills

Unrealistic expectation for self, infant, partner

Limited cognitive functioning

Lack of knowledge about child development

Inability to recognize and act on infant cues

Low educational level or attainment

Poor communication skills

Lack of cognitive readiness for parenthood

Preference for physical punishment

Physiological

Physical illness

Infant or Child

- Premature birth
- Illness
- Prolonged separation from parent
- Not desired gender
- Attention deficit hyperactivity disorder
- Difficult temperament
- Separation from parent at birth
- Lack of goodness of fit (temperament) with parental expectations
- Unplanned or unwanted child
- Handicapping condition or developmental delay
- Multiple births
- Altered perceptual abilities

Psychological

- History of substance abuse or dependencies
- Disability
- Depression
- Difficult labor and/or delivery
- Young age, especially adolescent
- History of mental illness
- High number or closely spaced pregnancies
- Sleep deprivation or disruption
- Lack of, or late, prenatal care
- Separation from infant/ child

Note. It is important to reaffirm that adjustment to parenting in general is a normal maturational process that elicits nursing behaviors to prevent potential problems and to promote health.

RISK FOR IMPAIRED PARENTING*
(1978, 1998)

Definition *Risk for inability of the primary caretaker to create, maintain, or regain an environment that promotes the optimum growth and development of the child*

Risk Factors

Social

Marital conflict, declining satisfaction

History of being abused

Poor problem-solving skills

Role strain/overload

Social isolation

Legal difficulties

Lack of access to resources

Lack of value of parenthood

Relocation

Poverty

Poor home environment

Lack of family cohesiveness

Lack of or poor parental role model

Father of child not involved

History of being abusive

Financial difficulties

Low self-esteem

Lack of resources

Unplanned or unwanted pregnancy

Inadequate child care arrangements

Maladaptive coping strategies

Low socioeconomic class

Lack of transportation

Change in family unit

Unemployment or job problems

Single parent

Lack of social support network

Inability to put child's needs before own

Stress

Knowledge

Low educational level or attainment

Unrealistic expectations of child

Lack of knowledge about parenting skills

Poor communication skills

Preference for physical punishment

* Formerly "Risk for Altered Parenting"

Inability to recognize and act on infant cues

Low cognitive functioning

Lack of knowledge about child health maintenance

Lack of knowledge about child development

Lack of cognitive readiness for parenthood

Physiological

Physical illness

Infant or Child

Multiple births

Handicapping condition or developmental delay

Illness

Altered perceptual abilities

Lack of goodness of fit (temperament) with parental expectations

Unplanned or unwanted child

Premature birth

Not gender desired

Difficult temperament

Attention deficit hyperactivity disorder

Prolonged separation from parent

Separation from parent at birth

Psychological

Separation from infant/child

High number or closely spaced children

Disability

Sleep deprivation or disruption

Difficult labor and/or delivery

Young age, especially adolescent

Depression

History of mental illness

Lack of, or late, prenatal care

History of substance abuse or dependence

P

Note. It is important to reaffirm that adjustment to parenting in general is a normal maturational process that elicits nursing behaviors to prevent potential problems and to promote health.

RISK FOR PERIPHERAL NEUROVASCULAR DYSFUNCTION
(1992)

Definition *At risk for disruption in circulation, sensation, or motion of an extremity*

Risk Factors

Trauma
Vascular obstruction
Orthopedic surgery
Fractures
Burns
Mechanical compression
  (e.g., tourniquet, cane,
  cast, brace, dressing,
  restraint)
Immobilization

P

RISK FOR POISONING
(1980)

Definition *At accentuated risk of accidental exposure to, or ingestion of, drugs or dangerous products in doses sufficient to cause poisoning*

Risk Factors

External

Unprotected contact with heavy metals or chemicals

Medicines stored in unlocked cabinets accessible to children or confused people

Presence of poisonous vegetation

Presence of atmospheric pollutants

Paint, lacquer, etc., in poorly ventilated areas or without effective protection

Flaking, peeling paint or plaster in presence of young children

Chemical contamination of food and water

Availability of illicit drugs potentially contaminated by poisonous additives

Large supplies of drugs in house

Dangerous products placed or stored within reach of children or confused people

Internal

Verbalization that occupational setting is without adequate safeguards

Reduced vision

Lack of safety or drug education

Lack of proper precaution

Insufficient finances

Cognitive or emotional difficulties

POST-TRAUMA SYNDROME
(1986, 1998)

Definition *Sustained maladaptive response to a traumatic, overwhelming event*

Defining Characteristics

- Avoidance
- Repression
- Difficulty in concentrating
- Grief
- Intrusive thoughts
- Neurosensory irritability
- Palpitations
- Enuresis (in children)
- Anger and/or rage
- Intrusive dreams
- Nightmares
- Aggression
- Hypervigilant
- Exaggerated startle response
- Hopelessness
- Altered mood states
- Shame
- Panic attacks
- Alienation
- Denial
- Horror
- Substance abuse
- Depression
- Anxiety
- Guilt
- Fear
- Gastric irritability
- Detachment
- Psychogenic amnesia
- Irritability
- Numbing
- Compulsive behavior
- Flashbacks
- Headaches

Related Factors

Events outside the range of usual human experience

Physical and psychosocial abuse

Tragic occurrence involving multiple deaths

Epidemics

Sudden destruction of one's home or community

Being held prisoner of war or criminal victimization (torture)

Wars

Rape

Natural and/or man-
made disasters
Serious accidents
Witnessing mutilation,
violent death, or other
horrors

Serious threat or injury to
self or loved ones
Industrial and motor
vehicle accidents
Military combat

P

RISK FOR POST-TRAUMA SYNDROME
(1998)

Definition *At risk for sustained maladaptive response to a traumatic, overwhelming event*

Risk Factors

Exaggerated sense of responsibility
Perception of event
Survivor's role in the event
Occupation (e.g., police, fire, rescue, corrections, emergency room staff, mental health worker)

Displacement from home
Inadequate social support
Nonsupportive environment
Diminished ego strength
Duration of the event

P

POWERLESSNESS
(1982)

Definition *Perception that one's own action will not significantly affect an outcome; a perceived lack of control over a current situation or immediate happening*

Defining Characteristics

Low

- Expressions of uncertainty about fluctuating energy levels
- Passivity

Moderate

- Nonparticipation in care or decision making when opportunities are provided
- Resentment, anger, guilt
- Reluctance to express true feelings
- Passivity
- Dependence on others that may result in irritability
- Fearing alienation from caregivers
- Expressions of dissatisfaction and frustration over inability to perform previous tasks/activities

- Expression of doubt regarding role performance
- Does not monitor progress
- Does not defend self-care practices when challenged
- Inability to seek information regarding care

Severe

- Verbal expressions of having no control
  - Over self-care
  - Or influence over situation
  - Or influence over outcome
- Apathy
- Depression over physical deterioration that occurs despite patient compliance with regimens

Related Factors

Healthcare environment
Illness-related regimen
Interpersonal interaction
Lifestyle of helplessness

RISK FOR POWERLESSNESS
(2000)

Definition *At risk for perceived lack of control over a situation and/or one's ability to significantly affect an outcome*

Risk Factors

Physiological

Chronic or acute illness (hospitalization, intubation, ventilator, suctioning)

Acute injury or progressive debilitating disease process (e.g., spinal cord injury, multiple sclerosis)

Aging (e.g., decreased physical strength, decreased mobility)

Dying

Psychosocial

Lack of knowledge of illness or healthcare system

Lifestyle of dependency with inadequate coping patterns

Absence of integrality (e.g., essence of power)

Decreased self-esteem

Low or unstable body image

P

INEFFECTIVE PROTECTION*
(1990)

Definition *Decrease in the ability to guard self from internal or external threats such as illness or injury*

Defining Characteristics

- Maladaptive stress response
- Neurosensory alteration
- Impaired healing
- Deficient immunity
- Altered clotting
- Dyspnea
- Insomnia
- Weakness
- Restlessness
- Pressure ulcers
- Perspiring
- Itching
- Immobility
- Chilling
- Fatigue
- Disorientation
- Cough
- Anorexia

Related Factors

Abnormal blood profiles (e.g., leukopenia, thrombocytopenia, anemia, coagulation)
Inadequate nutrition
Extremes of age
Drug therapies (e.g., antineoplastic, corticosteroid, immune, anticoagulant, thrombolytic)

Alcohol abuse
Treatments (e.g., surgery, radiation)
Diseases such as cancer and immune disorders

P

---

* *Formerly "Altered Protection"*

Rape-Trauma Syndrome
(1980, 1998)

Definition *Sustained maladaptive response to a forced, violent sexual penetration against the victim's will and consent*

Defining Characteristics

- Disorganization
- Change in relationships
- Confusion
- Physical trauma (e.g., bruising, tissue irritation)
- Suicide attempts
- Denial
- Guilt
- Paranoia
- Humiliation
- Embarrassment
- Aggression
- Muscle tension and/or spasms
- Mood swings
- Dependence
- Powerlessness
- Nightmares and sleep disturbances
- Sexual dysfunction
- Revenge
- Phobias
- Loss of self-esteem
- Inability to make decisions
- Dissociative disorders
- Self-blame
- Hyperalertness
- Vulnerability
- Substance abuse
- Depression
- Helplessness
- Anger
- Anxiety
- Agitation
- Shame
- Shock
- Fear

Related Factors

Rape

Note. This syndrome includes the following three sub-components: Rape-Trauma, Compound Reaction, and Silent Reaction. In this text each appears as a separate diagnosis.

Rape-Trauma Syndrome: Compound Reaction
(1980)

Definition *Forced violent sexual penetration against the victim's will and consent. The trauma syndrome that develops from this attack or attempted attack includes an acute phase of disorganization of the victim's lifestyle and a long-term process of reorganization of lifestyle.*

Defining Characteristics

- Change in lifestyle (e.g., changes in residence, dealing with repetitive nightmares and phobias, seeking family support, seeking social network support in long-term phase)
- Emotional reaction (e.g., anger, embarrassment, fear of physical violence and death, humiliation, revenge, self-blame in acute phase)
- Multiple physical symptoms (e.g., gastrointestinal irritability, genitourinary discomfort, muscle tension, sleep pattern disturbance in acute phase)
- Reactivated symptoms of such previous conditions (i.e., physical illness, psychiatric illness in acute phase)
- Reliance on alcohol/drugs (acute phase)

Related Factors

To be developed

R

Note. This syndrome includes the following three subcomponents: Rape-Trauma, Compound Reaction, and Silent Reaction. In this text each appears as a separate diagnosis.

Rape-trauma syndrome: silent reaction
(1980)

Definition *Forced violent sexual penetration against the victim's will and consent. The trauma syndrome that develops from this attack or attempted attack includes an acute phase of disorganization of the victim's lifestyle and a long-term process of reorganization of lifestyle.*

Defining Characteristics

- Increased anxiety during interview (i.e., blocking of associations, long periods of silence, minor stuttering, physical distress)
- Sudden onset of phobic reactions
- No verbalization of the occurrence of rape
- Abrupt changes in relationships with men
- Increase in nightmares
- Pronounced changes in sexual behavior

Related Factors

To be developed

Note. This syndrome includes the following three subcomponents: Rape-Trauma, Compound Reaction, and Silent Reaction. In this text each appears as a separate diagnosis.

R

Relocation Stress Syndrome
(1992, 2000)

Definition *Physiological and/or psychosocial disturbance following transfer from one environment to another*

Defining Characteristics

- Temporary or permanent move
- Voluntary/involuntary move
- Aloneness, alienation, loneliness
- Depression
- Anxiety (e.g., separation)
- Sleep disturbance
- Withdrawal
- Anger
- Loss of identity, self-worth, or self-esteem
- Increased verbalization of needs, unwillingness to move, or concern over relocation
- Increased physical symptoms/illness (e.g., gastrointestinal disturbance, weight change)
- Dependency
- Insecurity
- Pessimism
- Frustration
- Worry
- Fear

Related Factors

Unpredictability of experience
Isolation from family/friends
Past, concurrent, and recent losses
Feelings of powerlessness
Lack of adequate support system/group
Lack of predeparture counseling
Passive coping
Impaired psychosocial health
Language barrier
Deceased health status

R

RISK FOR RELOCATION STRESS SYNDROME
(2000)

Definition *At risk for physiological and/or psychosocial disturbance following transfer from one environment to another*

Defining Characteristics

- Moderate to high degree of environmental change (e.g., physical, ethnic, cultural)
- Temporary and/or permanent moves
- Voluntary/involuntary move
- Lack of adequate support system/group
- Feelings of powerlessness
- Moderate mental competence (e.g., alert enough to experience changes)
- Unpredictability of experiences
- Decreased psychosocial or physical health status
- Lack of predeparture counseling
- Passive coping
- Past, current, recent losses

R

INEFFECTIVE ROLE PERFORMANCE*
(1978, 1996, 1998)

Definition *Patterns of behavior and self-expression that do not match the environmental context, norms, and expectations*

Defining Characteristics

- Change in self-perception of role
- Role denial
- Inadequate external support for role enactment
- Inadequate adaptation to change or transition
- System conflict
- Change in usual patterns of responsibility
- Discrimination
- Domestic violence
- Harassment
- Uncertainty
- Altered role perceptions
- Role strain
- Inadequate self-management
- Role ambivalence
- Pessimistic attitude
- Inadequate motivation
- Inadequate confidence
- Inadequate role competency and skills
- Inadequate knowledge
- Inappropriate developmental expectations
- Role conflict
- Role confusion
- Powerlessness
- Inadequate coping
- Anxiety or depression
- Role overload
- Change in other's perception of role
- Change in capacity to resume role
- Role dissatisfaction
- Inadequate opportunities for role enactment

Related Factors
Social

Inadequate or inappropriate linkage with the healthcare system
Job schedule demands

Young age, developmental level
Lack of rewards
Poverty

continued

R

* Formerly "Altered Role Performance"

Ineffective Role Performance, *continued*

Family conflict
Inadequate support
system
Inadequate role socializa-
tion (e.g., role model,
expectations,
responsibilities)
Low socioeconomic status
Stress and conflict
Domestic violence
Lack of resources

Knowledge

Inadequate role prepara-
tion (e.g., role transi-
tion, skill rehearsal,
validation)
Lack of knowledge about
role, role skills
Role transition
Lack of opportunity for
role rehearsal
Developmental transitions
Unrealistic role
expectations
Education attainment level
Lack of or inadequate
role model

Physiological

Inadequate/inappropri-
ate linkage with health-
care system
Substance abuse
Mental illness
Body image alteration
Physical illness
Cognitive deficits
Health alterations (e.g.,
physical health, body
image, self-esteem,
mental health, psy-
chosocial health, cogni-
tion, learning style,
neurological health)
Depression
Low self-esteem
Pain
Fatigue

R

Note. There is a typology of roles: Sociopersonal (friend-
ship, family, marital, parenting, community), home
management, intimacy (sexuality, relationship building), leisure/exercise/recreation, self-management,
socialization (developmental transitions), community
contributor, and religious.

BATHING/HYGIENE **S**ELF-CARE DEFICIT
(1980, 1998)

Definition *Impaired ability to perform or complete bathing/hygiene activities for oneself*

Defining Characteristics

- Inability to
    - Wash body or body parts
    - Obtain or get to water source
    - Regulate temperature or flow of bath water
    - Get bath supplies
    - Dry body
    - Get in and out of bathroom

Related Factors

Decreased or lack of motivation

Weakness and tiredness

Severe anxiety

Inability to perceive body part or spatial relationship

Perceptual or cognitive impairment

Pain

Neuromuscular impairment

Musculoskeletal impairment

Environmental barriers

Note. See suggested Functional Level Classification under *Impaired Physical Mobility* (p. 118).

DRESSING/GROOMING SELF-CARE DEFICIT
(1980, 1998)

Definition *Impaired ability to perform or complete dressing and grooming activities for self*

Defining Characteristics

- Impaired ability to
  - Put on or take off necessary items of clothing
  - Fasten clothing
  - Obtain or replace articles of clothing
- Inability to
  - Put on clothing on upper body
  - Put on clothing on lower body

  - Choose clothing
  - Use assistive devices
  - Use zippers
  - Remove clothes
  - Put on socks
  - Maintain appearance at a satisfactory level
  - Pick up clothing
  - Put on shoes

Related Factors

Decreased or lack of motivation
Pain
Severe anxiety
Perceptual or cognitive impairment
Weakness or tiredness

Neuromuscular impairment
Musculoskeletal impairment
Discomfort
Environmental barriers

S

Note. See suggested Functional Level Classification under *Impaired Physical Mobility* (p. 118).

FEEDING Self-CARE DEFICIT
(1980, 1998)

Definition   *Impaired ability to perform or complete feeding activities*

Defining Characteristics

- Inability to
  - Swallow food
  - Prepare food for ingestion
  - Handle utensils
  - Chew food
  - Use assistive device
  - Get food onto utensil
  - Open containers
  - Ingest food safely
  - Manipulate food in mouth
  - Bring food from a receptacle to the mouth
  - Complete a meal
  - Ingest food in a socially acceptable manner
  - Pick up cup or glass
  - Ingest sufficient food

Related Factors

Weakness or tiredness
Severe anxiety
Neuromuscular impairment
Pain
Perceptual or cognitive impairment

Discomfort
Environmental barriers
Decreased or lack of motivation
Musculoskeletal impairments

Note. See suggested Functional Level Classification under *Impaired Physical Mobility* (p. 118).

S

TOILETING SELF-CARE DEFICIT
(1980, 1998)

Definition *Impaired ability to perform or complete own toileting activities*

Defining Characteristics

- Inability to
  - Get to toilet or commode
  - Sit on or rise from toilet or commode
  - Manipulate clothing for toileting
  - Carry out proper toilet hygiene
  - Flush toilet or commode

Related Factors

Environmental barriers
Weakness or tiredness
Decreased or lack of motivation
Severe anxiety
Impaired mobility status
Impaired transfer ability
Musculoskeletal impairment
Neuromuscular impairment
Pain
Perceptual or cognitive impairment

Note. See suggested Functional Level Classification under *Impaired Physical Mobility* (p. 118).

S

CHRONIC LOW SELF-ESTEEM
(1988, 1996)

Definition   *Long-standing negative self-evaluation/feelings about self or self-capabilities*

Defining Characteristics

- Rationalizes away/rejects positive feedback and exaggerates negative feedback about self (long standing or chronic)
- Self-negating verbalization (long standing or chronic)
- Hesitant to try new things/situations (long standing or chronic)
- Expressions of shame/ guilt (long standing or chronic)

- Evaluates self as unable to deal with events (long standing or chronic)
- Lack of eye contact
- Nonassertive/passive
- Frequent lack of success in work or other life events
- Excessively seeks reassurance
- Overly conforming, dependent on others' opinions
- Indecisive

Related Factors

To be developed

S

SITUATIONAL LOW SELF-ESTEEM
(1988, 1996, 2000)

Definition *Development of a negative perception of self-worth in response to a current situation (specify)*

Defining Characteristics

- Verbally reports current situational challenge to self-worth
- Self-negating verbalizations
- Indecisive, nonassertive behavior
- Evaluation of self as unable to deal with situations or events
- Expressions of helplessness and uselessness

Related Factors

Developmental changes (specify)
Disturbed body image
Functional impairment (specify)
Loss (specify)
Social role changes (specify)

Lack of recognition/ rewards
Behavior inconsistent with values
Failures/rejections

S

RISK FOR SITUATIONAL LOW Sᴇʟꜰ-ᴇꜱᴛᴇᴇᴍ
(2000)

Definition *At risk for developing negative perception of self-worth in response to a current situation (specify)*

Risk Factors

Developmental changes (specify)

Disturbed body image

Functional impairment (specify)

Loss (specify)

Social role changes (specify)

History of learned helplessness

History of abuse, neglect, or abandonment

Unrealistic self-expectations

Behavior inconsistent with values

Lack of recognition/ rewards

Failures/rejections

Decreased power/control over environment

Physical illness (specify)

S

SELF-MUTILATION
(2000)

Definition *Deliberate self-injurious behavior causing tissue damage with the intent of causing nonfatal injury to attain relief of tension*

Defining Characteristics

- Cuts/scratches on body
- Picking at wounds
- Self-inflicted burns (e.g., eraser, cigarette)
- Ingestion/inhalation of harmful substances/objects
- Biting
- Abrading
- Severing
- Insertion of object(s) into body orifice(s)
- Hitting
- Constricting a body part

Related Factors

Psychotic state (command hallucinations)

Inability to express tension verbally

Childhood sexual abuse

Violence between parental figures

Family divorce

Family alcoholism

Family history of self-destructive behaviors

Adolescence

Peers who self-mutilate

Isolation from peers

Perfectionism

Substance abuse

Eating disorders

Sexual identity crisis

Low or unstable self-esteem

Low or unstable body image

Labile behavior (mood swings)

History of inability to plan solutions or see long-term consequences

Use of manipulation to obtain nurturing relationship with others

Chaotic/disturbed interpersonal relationships

Emotionally disturbed; battered child

Feels threatened with actual or potential loss of significant relationship (e.g., loss of parent/parental relationship)

Experiences dissociation or depersonalization

Mounting tension that is intolerable

Impulsivity

Inadequate coping

Irresistible urge to cut/damage self

Needs quick reduction of stress

Childhood illness or surgery

Foster, group, or institutional care

Incarceration

Character disorder

Borderline personality disorder

Developmentally delayed or autistic individual

History of self-injurious behavior

Feelings of depression, rejection, self-hatred, separation anxiety, guilt, depersonalization

Poor parent-adolescent communication

Lack of family confidant

S

RISK FOR SELF-MUTILATION
(1992, 2000)

Definition *At risk for deliberate self-injurious behavior causing tissue damage with the intent of causing nonfatal injury to attain relief of tension*

Risk Factors

Psychotic state (command hallucinations)

Inability to express tension verbally

Childhood sexual abuse

Violence between parental figures

Family divorce

Family alcoholism

Family history of self-destructive behaviors

Adolescence

Peers who self-mutilate

Isolation from peers

Perfectionism

Substance abuse

Eating disorders

Sexual identity crisis

Low or unstable self-esteem

Low or unstable body image

History of inability to plan solutions or see long-term consequences

Use of manipulation to obtain nurturing relationship with others

Chaotic/disturbed interpersonal relationships

Emotionally disturbed and/or battered children

Feels threatened with actual or potential loss of significant relationship

Loss of parent/parental relationships

Experiences dissociation or depersonalization

Experiences mounting tension that is intolerable

Impulsivity

Inadequate coping

Experiences irresistible urge to cut/damage self

Needs quick reduction of stress

Childhood illness or surgery

Foster, group, or institutional care

Incarceration

Character disorders

Borderline personality disorders

Loss of control over problem-solving situations

Developmentally delayed or autistic individuals

History of self-injurious behavior

Feelings of depression, rejection, self-hatred, separation anxiety, guilt, and depersonalization

S

DISTURBED SENSORY PERCEPTION (Specify: Visual, Auditory, Kinesthetic, Gustatory, Tactile, Olfactory)*
(1978, 1980, 1998)

Definition *Change in the amount or patterning of incoming stimuli accompanied by a diminished, exaggerated, distorted, or impaired response to such stimuli*

Defining Characteristics

- Poor concentration
- Auditory distortions
- Change in usual response to stimuli
- Restlessness
- Reported or measured change in sensory acuity
- Irritability
- Disoriented in time, in place, or with people
- Change in problem-solving abilities
- Change in behavior pattern
- Altered communication patterns
- Hallucinations
- Visual distortions

Related Factors

Altered sensory perception
Excessive environmental stimuli
Psychological stress
Altered sensory reception, transmission, and/or integration
Insufficient environmental stimuli

Biochemical imbalances for sensory distortion (e.g., illusions, hallucinations)
Electrolyte imbalance
Biochemical imbalance

* Formerly "Sensory/Perceptual Alterations"

Sexual dysfunction
(1980)

Definition *Change in sexual function that is viewed as unsatisfying, unrewarding, inadequate*

Defining Characteristics
- Change of interest in self and others
- Conflicts involving values
- Inability to achieve desired satisfaction
- Verbalization of problem
- Alteration in relationship with significant other
- Alteration in achieving sexual satisfaction
- Actual or perceived limitations imposed by disease and/or therapy
- Seeking confirmation of desirability
- Alterations in achieving perceived sex role

Related Factors
Misinformation or lack of knowledge
Vulnerability
Values conflict
Psychosocial abuse (e.g., harmful relationships)
Physical abuse
Lack of privacy
Ineffectual or absent role models
Altered body structure of function (e.g., pregnancy, recent childbirth, drugs, surgery, anomalies, disease process, trauma, radiation)
Lack of significant other
Biopsychosocial alteration of sexuality

S

INEFFECTIVE SEXUALITY PATTERNS*
(1986)

Definition *Expressions of concern regarding own sexuality*

Defining Characteristics
• Reported difficulties, limitations, or changes in sexual behaviors or activities

Related Factors
Lack of significant other

Conflicts with sexual orientation or variant preferences

Fear of pregnancy or of acquiring a sexually transmitted disease

Impaired relationship with a significant other

Ineffective or absent role models

Knowledge/skill deficit about alternative responses to health-related transitions, altered body function or structure, illness or medical treatment

Lack of privacy

S

---

* *Formerly "Altered Sexuality Patterns"*

IMPAIRED SKIN INTEGRITY
(1975, 1998)

Definition *Altered epidermis and/or dermis*

Defining Characteristics
- Invasion of body structures
- Destruction of skin layers (dermis)
- Disruption of skin surface (epidermis)

Related Factors

External

Hyperthermia or hypothermia
Chemical substance
Humidity
Mechanical factors (e.g., shearing forces, pressure, restraint)
Physical immobilization
Radiation
Extremes in age
Moisture
Medications

Internal

Altered metabolic state
Skeletal prominence
Immunological deficit
Developmental factors
Altered sensation
Altered nutritional state (e.g., obesity, emaciation)
Altered pigmentation
Altered circulation
Alterations in turgor (changes in elasticity)
Altered fluid status

S

RISK FOR IMPAIRED SKIN INTEGRITY
(1975, 1998)

Definition   *At risk for skin being adversely altered*

Risk Factors

External

Radiation
Physical immobilization
Mechanical factors (e.g., shearing forces, pressure, restraint)
Hypothermia or hyperthermia
Humidity
Chemical substance
Excretions and/or secretions
Moisture
Extremes of age

Internal

Medication
Skeletal prominence
Immunologic factors
Developmental factors
Altered sensation
Altered pigmentation
Altered metabolic state
Altered circulation
Alterations in skin turgor (changes in elasticity)
Alterations in nutritional state (e.g., obesity, emaciation)
Psychogenetic

Note. Risk should be determined by the use of a risk assessment tool (e.g., Braden Scale).

S

SLEEP DEPRIVATION
(1998)

Definition *Prolonged periods of time without sleep (sustained natural, periodic suspension of relative consciousness)*

Defining Characteristics

- Daytime drowsiness
- Decreased ability to function
- Malaise
- Tiredness
- Lethargy
- Restlessness
- Irritability
- Heightened sensitivity to pain
- Listlessness
- Apathy
- Slowed reaction
- Inability to concentrate
- Perceptual disorders (e.g., disturbed body sensation, delusions, feeling afloat)
- Hallucinations
- Acute confusion
- Transient paranoia
- Agitated or combative
- Anxious
- Mild, fleeting nystagmus
- Hand tremors

Related Factors

Prolonged physical discomfort

Prolonged psychological discomfort

Sustained inadequate sleep hygiene

Prolonged use of pharmacologic or dietary antisoporifics

Aging-related sleep stage shifts

Sustained circadian asynchrony

Inadequate daytime activity

Sustained environmental stimulation

Sustained unfamiliar or uncomfortable sleep environment

Non-sleep-inducing parenting practices

Sleep apnea

Periodic limb movement (e.g., restless leg syndrome, nocturnal myoclonus)

Sundowner's syndrome

Narcolepsy

continued

S

Sleep Deprivation, *continued*

Idiopathic central nervous
  system hypersomnolence
Sleep walking
Sleep terror
Sleep-related enuresis

Nightmares
Familial sleep paralysis
Sleep-related painful
  erections
Dementia

S

DISTURBED SLEEP PATTERN*
(1980, 1998)

Definition *Time-limited disruption of sleep (natural, periodic suspension of consciousness) amount and quality*

Defining Characteristics

- Prolonged awakenings
- Sleep maintenance insomnia
- Self-induced impairment of normal pattern
- Sleep onset >30 minutes
- Early morning insomnia
- Awakening earlier or later than desired
- Verbal complaints of difficulty falling asleep
- Verbal complaints of not feeling well-rested
- Increased proportion of Stage 1 sleep
- Less than age-normed total sleep time

- Dissatisfaction with sleep
- Three or more nighttime awakenings
- Decreased proportion of Stages 3 and 4 sleep (e.g., hyporesponsiveness, excess sleepiness, decreased motivation)
- Decreased proportion of REM sleep (e.g., REM rebound, hyperactivity, emotional lability, agitation and impulsivity, atypical polysomnographic features)
- Decreased ability to function

Related Factors

Psychological

Ruminative presleep thoughts
Daytime activity pattern
Thinking about home
Body temperature
Temperament
Dietary

Childhood onset
Inadequate sleep hygiene
Sustained use of anti-sleep agents
Circadian asynchrony
Frequently changing sleep–wake schedule
Depression

continued

* *Formerly "Sleep Pattern Disturbance"*

Disturbed Sleep Pattern, *continued*

Loneliness
Frequent travel across time zones
Daylight/darkness exposure
Grief
Anticipation
Shift work
Delayed or advanced sleep phase syndrome
Loss of sleep partner, life change
Preoccupation with trying to sleep
Periodic gender-related hormonal shifts
Biochemical agents
Fear
Separation from significant others
Social schedule inconsistent with chronotype
Aging-related sleep shifts
Anxiety
Medications
Fear of insomnia
Maladaptive conditioned wakefulness
Fatigue
Boredom

Environmental

Noise
Lighting

Unfamiliar sleep furnishings
Ambient temperature, humidity
Other-generated awakening
Excessive stimulation
Physical restraint
Lack of sleep privacy/control
Interruptions for therapeutics, monitoring, lab tests
Sleep partner
Noxious odors

Parental

Mother's sleep-wake pattern
Parent-infant interaction
Mother's emotional support

Physiological

Urinary urgency, incontinence
Fever
Nausea
Stasis of secretions
Shortness of breath
Position
Gastroesophageal reflux

IMPAIRED SOCIAL INTERACTION
(1986)

Definition *Insufficient or excessive quantity or ineffective quality of social exchange*

Defining Characteristics

- Verbalized or observed inability to receive or communicate a satisfying sense of belonging, caring, interest, or shared history
- Verbalized or observed discomfort in social situations
- Observed use of unsuccessful social interaction behaviors
- Dysfunctional interaction with peers, family and/or others
- Family report of change of style or pattern of interaction

Related Factors

Knowledge/skill deficit about ways to enhance mutuality
Therapeutic isolation
Sociocultural dissonance
Limited physical mobility

Environmental barriers
Communication barriers
Altered thought processes
Absence of available significant others or peers
Self-concept disturbance

S

SOCIAL ISOLATION
(1982)

Definition *Aloneness experienced by the individual and perceived as imposed by others and as a negative or threatening state*

Defining Characteristics

Objective
- Absence of supportive significant other(s) (family, friends, group)
- Projects hostility in voice, behavior
- Withdrawn
- Uncommunicative
- Shows behavior unaccepted by dominant cultural group
- Seeks to be alone or exists in a subculture
- Repetitive, meaningless actions
- Preoccupation with own thoughts
- No eye contact
- Inappropriate or immature activities for developmental age/stage
- Evidence of physical/mental handicap or altered state of wellness
- Sad, dull affect

Subjective
- Expresses feelings of aloneness imposed by others
- Expresses feelings of rejection
- Inappropriate or immature interests for developmental age/stage
- Inadequate or absent significant purpose in life
- Inability to meet expectations of others
- Expresses values acceptable to the subculture but unacceptable to the dominant cultural group
- Expresses interests inappropriate to the developmental age/stage
- Experiences feelings of differences from others
- Insecurity in public

S

Related Factors

Alterations in mental
  status
Inability to engage in
  satisfying personal
  relationships
Unaccepted social values
Unaccepted social
  behavior
Inadequate personal
  resources

Immature interests
Factors contributing to
  the absence of satisfying
  personal relationships
  (e.g., delay in accom-
  plishing developmental
  tasks)
Alterations in physical
  appearance
Altered state of wellness

S

CHRONIC SORROW
(1998)

Definition *Cyclical, recurring, and potentially progressive pattern of pervasive sadness experienced (by a parent, caregiver, individual with chronic illness or disability) in response to continual loss, throughout the trajectory of an illness or disability*

Defining Characteristics

- Expresses periodic, recurrent feelings of sadness
- Feelings that vary in intensity, are periodic, may progress and intensify over time, and may interfere with the client's ability to reach his/her highest level of personal and social well-being
- Expresses one or more of the following feelings: anger, being misunderstood, confusion, depression, disappointment, emptiness, fear, frustration, guilt/self-blame, helplessness, hopelessness, loneliness, low self-esteem, recurring loss, overwhelmed

Related Factors

Death of a loved one
Experiences chronic physical or mental illness or disability (e.g., mental retardation, multiple sclerosis, prematurity, spina bifida or other birth defects, chronic mental illness, infertility, cancer, Parkinson's disease)

Experiences one or more trigger events (e.g., crises in management of the illness, crises related to developmental stages, missed opportunities or milestones that bring comparisons with developmental, social, or personal norms)
Unending caregiving as a constant reminder of loss

S

Spiritual Distress
(1978)

Definition *Disruption in the life principle that pervades a person's entire being and that integrates and transcends one's biological and psychosocial nature*

Defining Characteristics

- Expresses concern with meaning of life/death and/or belief systems
- Questions moral/ethical implications of therapeutic regimen
- Describes nightmares/sleep disturbances
- Verbalizes inner conflict about beliefs
- Verbalizes concern about relationship with deity
- Unable to participate in usual religious practices
- Seeks spiritual assistance
- Questions meaning of suffering
- Questions meaning of own existence
- Displacement of anger toward religious representatives
- Anger toward God
- Alteration in behavior/mood evidenced by anger, crying, withdrawal, preoccupation, anxiety, hostility, apathy, etc.
- Gallows humor (inappropriate humor in a grave situation)

Related Factors

Challenged belief and value system (e.g., due to moral/ethical implications of therapy, intense suffering)

Separation from religious/cultural ties

S

RISK FOR SPIRITUAL DISTRESS
(1998)

Definition *At risk for an altered sense of harmonious connectedness with all of life and the universe in which dimensions that transcend and empower the self may be disrupted*

Risk Factors

Energy-consuming anxiety
Low self-esteem
Mental illness
Physical illness
Blocks to self-love
Poor relationships
Physical or psychological
  stress
Substance abuse
Loss of loved one
Natural disasters
Situational losses
Maturational losses
Inability to forgive

S

READINESS FOR ENHANCED Spiritual WELL-BEING*
(1994)

Definition *Process of developing/unfolding of mystery through harmonious interconnectedness that springs from inner strengths*

Defining Characteristics

Inner Strengths

- Inner core
- Transcendence
- Self-consciousness
- Unifying force
- Sense of awareness
- Sacred source

Unfolding Mystery

- One's experience about life's purpose and meaning, mystery, uncertainty, and struggles

Harmonious Interconnectedness

- Harmony with self, others, Higher Power/God, and the environment
- Relatedness with self, others, Higher Power/God, and the environment
- Connectedness with self, others, Higher Power/God, and the environment

* *Formerly "Potential for Enhanced Spiritual Well-Being"*

RISK FOR SUFFOCATION
(1980)

Definition *Accentuated risk of accidental suffocation (inadequate air available for inhalation)*

Risk Factors

External

Vehicle warming in closed garage

Use of fuel-burning heaters not vented to outside

Smoking in bed

Children playing with plastic bags or inserting small objects into their mouths or noses

Propped bottle placed in an infant's crib

Pillow placed in an infant's crib

Person who eats large mouthfuls of food

Discarded or unused refrigerators or freezers without removed doors

Children left unattended in bathtubs or pools

Household gas leaks

Low-strung clothesline

Pacifier hung around infant's head

Internal

Reduced olfactory sensation

Reduced motor abilities

Cognitive or emotional difficulties

Disease or injury process

Lack of safety education

Lack of safety precautions

S

RISK FOR SUICIDE
(2000)

Definition   *At risk for self-inflicted, life-threatening injury*

Risk Factors

Behavioral

History of prior suicide
    attempt
Impulsiveness
Buying a gun
Stockpiling medicines
Making or changing a will
Giving away possessions
Sudden euphoric recovery
    from major depression
Marked changes in
    behavior, attitude,
    school performance

Verbal

Threats of killing oneself
States desire to die/end
    it all

Situational

Living alone
Retired
Relocation,
    institutionalization
Economic instability
Loss of autonomy/
    independence
Presence of gun in home

Adolescents living in
    nontraditional settings
    (e.g., juvenile detention
    center, prison, half-way
    house, group home)

Psychological

Family history of suicide
Alcohol and substance
    use/abuse
Psychiatric illness/
    disorder (e.g., depres-
    sion, schizophrenia,
    bipolar disorder)
Abuse in childhood
Guilt
Gay or lesbian youth

Demographic

Age: Elderly, young adult
    males, adolescents
Race: Caucasian, Native
    American
Gender: Male
Divorced, widowed

continued

S

Risk for Suicide, *continued*

Physical

Physical illness
Terminal illness
Chronic pain

Social

Loss of important
  relationship
Disrupted family life
Grief, bereavement

Poor support systems
Loneliness
Hopelessness
Helplessness
Social isolation
Legal or disciplinary
  problem
Cluster suicides

S

DELAYED SURGICAL RECOVERY
(1998)

Definition *Extension of the number of postoperative days required to initiate and perform activities that maintain life, health, and well-being*

Defining Characteristics

- Evidence of interrupted healing of surgical area (e.g., red, indurated, draining, immobilized)
- Loss of appetite with or without nausea
- Difficulty in moving about
- Requires help to complete self-care
- Fatigue
- Report of pain/discomfort
- Postpones resumption of work/employment activities
- Perception that more time is needed to recover

Related Factors

To be developed

S

IMPAIRED Swallowing
(1986, 1998)

Definition *Abnormal functioning of the swallowing mechanism associated with deficits in oral, pharyngeal, or esophageal structure or function*

Defining Characteristics

Pharyngeal Phase Impairment

- Altered head positions
- Inadequate laryngeal elevation
- Food refusal
- Unexplained fevers
- Delayed swallow
- Recurrent pulmonary infections
- Gurgly voice quality
- Nasal reflux
- Choking, coughing, or gagging
- Multiple swallows
- Abnormality in pharyngeal phase by swallow study

Esophageal Phase Impairment

- Heartburn or epigastric pain
- Acidic smelling breath
- Unexplained irritability surrounding mealtime
- Vomitus on pillow
- Repetitive swallowing or ruminating

- Regurgitation of gastric contents or wet burps
- Bruxism
- Nighttime coughing or awakening
- Observed evidence of difficulty in swallowing (e.g., stasis of food in oral cavity, coughing/choking)
- Hyperextension of head, arching during or after meals
- Abnormality in esophageal phase by swallow study
- Odynophagia
- Food refusal or volume limiting
- Complaints of "something stuck"
- Hematemesis
- Vomiting

Oral Phase Impairment

- Lack of tongue action to form bolus
- Weak suck resulting in inefficient nippling
- Incomplete lip closure

S

- Food pushed out of mouth
- Slow bolus formation
- Food falls from mouth
- Premature entry of bolus
- Inability to clear oral cavity
- Long meals with little consumption
- Nasal reflux
- Coughing, choking, gagging before a swallow
- Abnormality in oral phase of swallow study
- Piecemeal deglutition
- Lack of chewing
- Pooling in lateral sulci
- Sialorrhea or drooling

Related Factors

Congenital Deficits

Upper airway anomalies
Failure to thrive or protein energy malnutrition
Conditions with significant hypotonia
Respiratory disorders
History of tube feeding
Behavioral feeding problems
Self-injurious behavior
Neuromuscular impairment (e.g., decreased or absent gag reflex, decreased strength or excursion of muscles involved in mastication, perceptual impairment, facial paralysis)
Mechanical obstruction (e.g., edema, tracheostomy tube, tumor)
Congenital heart disease
Cranial nerve involvement

Neurological Problems

Upper airway anomalies
Laryngeal abnormalities
Achalasia
Gastroesophageal reflux disease
Acquired anatomic defects
Cerebral palsy
Internal or external traumas
Tracheal, laryngeal, esophageal defects
Traumatic head injury
Developmental delay
Nasal or nasopharyngeal cavity defects
Oral cavity or oropharynx abnormalities
Premature infants

S.

EFFECTIVE THERAPEUTIC REGIMEN MANAGEMENT*
(1994)

Definition *Pattern of regulating and integrating into daily living a program for treatment of illness and its sequelae that is satisfactory for meeting specific health goals*

Defining Characteristics

- Appropriate choices of daily activities for meeting the goals of a treatment or prevention program
- Illness symptoms within a normal range of expectation
- Verbalizes desire to manage the treatment of illness and prevention of sequelae
- Verbalizes intent to reduce risk factors for progression of illness and sequelae

Related Factors

To be developed

* Formerly "Effective Management of Therapeutic Regimen: Individual"

INEFFECTIVE THERAPEUTIC REGIMEN MANAGEMENT*
(1992)

Definition *Pattern of regulating and integrating into daily living a program for treatment of illness and the sequelae of illness that is unsatisfactory for meeting specific health goals*

Defining Characteristics

- Choices of daily living ineffective for meeting the goals of a treatment or prevention program
- Verbalizes that did not take action to reduce risk factors for progression of illness and sequelae
- Verbalizes desire to manage the treatment of illness and prevention of sequelae
- Verbalizes difficulty with regulation/integration of one or more prescribed regimens for prevention of complications and the treatment or illness or its effects
- Verbalizes that did not take action to include treatment regimens in daily routines

Related Factors

Perceived barriers
Social support deficit
Powerlessness
Perceived susceptibility
Perceived benefits
Mistrust of regimen and/or healthcare personnel
Knowledge deficit
Family patterns of health care
Family conflict

Excessive demands made on individual or family
Economic difficulties
Decisional conflicts
Complexity of therapeutic regimen
Complexity of healthcare system
Perceived seriousness
Inadequate number and types of cues to action

* *Formerly "Ineffective Management of Therapeutic Regimen: Individual"*

INEFFECTIVE COMMUNITY THERAPEUTIC REGIMEN MANAGEMENT*
(1994)

Definition *Pattern of regulating and integrating into community processes programs for treatment of illness and the sequelae of illness that are unsatisfactory for meeting health-related goals*

Defining Characteristics

- Illness symptoms above the norm expected for the number and type of population
- Unexpected acceleration of illness(es)
- Number of healthcare resources insufficient for the incidence or prevalence of illness(es)
- Deficits in advocates for aggregates
- Deficits in people and programs to be accountable for illness care of aggregates
- Deficits in community activities for secondary and tertiary prevention
- Unavailable healthcare resources for illness care

Related Factors

To be developed

T

* *Formerly "Ineffective Management of Therapeutic Regimen: Community"*

INEFFECTIVE FAMILY THERAPEUTIC REGIMEN MANAGEMENT*
(1994)

Definition *Pattern of regulating and integrating into family processes a program for treatment of illness and the sequelae of illness that is unsatisfactory for meeting specific health goals*

Defining Characteristics

- Inappropriate family activities for meeting the goals of a treatment or prevention program
- Acceleration of illness symptoms of a family member
- Lack of attention to illness and its sequelae
- Verbalizes difficulty with regulation/integration of one or more effects or prevention of complications
- Verbalizes desire to manage the treatment of illness and prevention of the sequelae
- Verbalizes that family did not take action to reduce risk factors for progression of illness and sequelae

Related Factors

Complexity of healthcare system
Complexity of therapeutic regimen
Decisional conflicts
Economic difficulties
Excessive demands made on individual or family
Family conflict

* Formerly "Ineffective Management of Therapeutic Regimen: Families"

INEFFECTIVE THERMOREGULATION
(1986)

Definition *Temperature fluctuation between hypothermia and hyperthermia*

Defining Characteristics

- Fluctuations in body temperature above and below the normal range
- Cool skin
- Cyanotic nail beds
- Flushed skin
- Hypertension
- Increased respiratory rate
- Pallor (moderate)
- Piloerection
- Reduction in body temperature below normal range
- Seizures/convulsions
- Shivering (mild)
- Slow capillary refill
- Tachycardia
- Warm to touch

Related Factors

Aging
Fluctuating environmental temperature
Immaturity
Trauma or illness

T

DISTURBED THOUGHT PROCESSES*
(1973, 1996)

Definition *Disruption in cognitive operations and activities*

Defining Characteristics

- Cognitive dissonance
- Memory deficit/problems
- Inaccurate interpretation of environment
- Hypovigilance
- Hypervigilance
- Distractibility
- Egocentricity
- Inappropriate nonreality-based thinking

Related Factors

To be developed

* *Formerly "Altered Thought Processes"*

IMPAIRED TISSUE INTEGRITY
(1986, 1998)

Definition *Damage to mucous membrane, corneal, integumentary, or subcutaneous tissues*

Defining Characteristics

- Damaged or destroyed tissue (e.g., cornea, mucous membrane, integumentary, subcutaneous)

Related Factors

Mechanical (e.g., pressure, shear, friction)
Radiation (including therapeutic radiation)
Nutritional deficit or excess
Thermal (temperature extremes)
Knowledge deficit
Irritants, chemical (including body excretions, secretions, medications)
Impaired physical mobility
Altered circulation
Fluid deficit or excess

T

INEFFECTIVE TISSUE PERFUSION (Specify Type: Renal, Cerebral, Cardiopulmonary, Gastrointestinal, Peripheral)*
(1980, 1998)

Definition *Decrease in oxygen resulting in the failure to nourish the tissues at the capillary level*

Defining Characteristics

Renal

- Altered blood pressure outside of acceptable parameters
- Hematuria
- Oliguria or anuria
- Elevation in BUN/ creatinine ratio

Gastrointestinal

- Hypoactive or absent bowel sounds
- Nausea
- Abdominal distention
- Abdominal pain or tenderness

Peripheral

- Edema
- Positive Homan's sign
- Altered skin characteristics (hair, nails, moisture)
- Weak or absent pulses
- Skin discolorations
- Skin temperature changes

- Altered sensations
- Claudication
- Blood pressure changes in extremities
- Bruits
- Delayed healing
- Diminished arterial pulsations
- Skin color pale on elevations, color does not return on lowering the leg

Cerebral

- Speech abnormalities
- Changes in pupillary reactions
- Extremity weakness or paralysis
- Altered mental status
- Difficulty in swallowing
- Changes in motor response
- Behavioral changes

continued

* *Formerly "Altered Tissue Perfusion"*

Ineffective Tissue Perfusion (Specify Type: Renal, Cerebral, Cardiopulmonary, Gastrointestinal, Peripheral), *continued*

Cardiopulmonary

- Altered respiratory rate outside of acceptable parameters
- Use of accessory muscles
- Capillary refill > 3 seconds
- Abnormal arterial blood gases
- Chest pain
- Sense of "impending doom"
- Bronchospasm
- Dyspnea
- Arrhythmias
- Nasal flaring
- Chest retraction

Related Factors

Hypovolemia
Hypervolemia
Interruption of flow, arterial
Exchange problems
Interruption of flow, venous
Mechanical reduction of venous and/or arterial blood flow
Hypoventilation

Impaired transport of the oxygen across alveolar and/or capillary membrane
Mismatch of ventilation with blood flow
Decreased hemoglobin concentration in blood
Enzyme poisoning
Altered affinity of hemoglobin for oxygen

T

IMPAIRED TRANSFER ABILITY
(1998)

Definition *Limitation of independent movement between two nearby surfaces*

Defining Characteristics

- Impaired ability to transfer
  - From bed to chair and chair to bed
  - On or off a toilet or commode
  - In and out of tub or shower
  - Between uneven levels
  - From chair to car or car to chair
  - From chair to floor or floor to chair
  - From standing to floor or floor to standing

Related Factors

To be developed

Note. Specify level of independence.

T

RISK FOR TRAUMA
(1980)

Definition *Accentuated risk of accidental tissue injury (e.g., wound, burn, fracture)*

Risk Factors

External

High-crime neighborhood and vulnerable clients

Pot handles facing toward front of stove

Knives stored uncovered

Inappropriate call-for-aid mechanisms for bed-resting client

Inadequately stored combustible or corrosives (e.g., matches, oily rags, lye)

Highly flammable children's toys or clothing

Obstructed passageways

High beds

Large icicles hanging from the roof

Nonuse or misuse of seat restraints

Overexposure to sun, sun lamps, radiotherapy

Overloaded electrical outlets

Overloaded fuse boxes

Play or work near vehicle pathways (e.g., driveways, lanes, railroad tracks)

Playing with fireworks or gunpowder

Guns or ammunition stored unlocked

Contact with rapidly moving machinery, industrial belts, or pulleys

Litter or liquid spills on floors or stairways

Defective appliances

Bathing in very hot water (e.g., unsupervised bathing of young children)

Bathtub without hand grip or antislip equipment

Children playing with matches, candles, cigarettes, sharp-edged toys

Children playing without gates at top of stairs

Children riding in the front seat in car

Delayed lighting of gas burner or oven

Contact with intense cold

Grease waste collected on stoves

Driving a mechanically unsafe vehicle

Driving after partaking of alcoholic beverages or drugs

Driving at excessive speeds

Entering unlighted rooms

Experimenting with chemical or gasoline

Exposure to dangerous machinery

Faulty electrical plugs

Frayed wires

Contact with acids or alkalis

Unsturdy or absent stair rails

Use of unsteady ladders or chairs

Use of cracked dishware or glasses

Wearing plastic apron or flowing clothes around open flame

Unscreened fires or heaters

Unsafe window protection in homes with young children

Sliding on coarse bed linen or struggling within bed restraints

Use of thin or worn potholders

Unanchored electric wires

Misuse of necessary headgear for motorized cyclists or young children carried on adult bicycles

Potential igniting of gas leaks

Unsafe road or road-crossing conditions

Slippery floors (e.g., wet or highly waxed)

Smoking in bed or near oxygen

Snow or ice collected on stairs, walkways

Unanchored rugs

Driving without necessary visual aids

Internal

Lack of safety education

Insufficient finances to purchase safety equipment or effect repairs

History of previous trauma

Lack of safety precautions

Poor vision

Reduced temperature and/or tactile sensation

Balancing difficulties

Cognitive or emotional difficulties

Reduced large or small muscle coordination

Weakness

Reduced hand-eye coordination

T

IMPAIRED URINARY ELIMINATION*
(1973)

Definition *Disturbance in urine elimination*

Defining Characteristics
- Incontinence
- Urgency
- Nocturia
- Hesitancy
- Frequency
- Dysuria
- Retention

Related Factors
Urinary tract infection
Anatomical obstruction
Multiple causality
Sensory motor impairment

U

* Formerly "Altered Urinary Elimination"

URINARY RETENTION
(1986)

Definition *Incomplete emptying of the bladder*

Defining Characteristics
- Bladder distention
- Small, frequent voiding or absence of urine output
- Dribbling
- Dysuria
- Overflow incontinence
- Residual urine
- Sensation of bladder fullness

Related Factors
Blockage
High urethral pressure caused by weak detrusor
Inhibition of reflex arc
Strong sphincter

U

IMPAIRED SPONTANEOUS VENTILATION*
(1992)

Definition *Decreased energy reserves result in an individual's inability to maintain breathing adequate to support life*

Defining Characteristics

- Dyspnea
- Increased metabolic rate
- Increased pCO_2
- Increased restlessness
- Increased heart rate
- Decreased tidal volume
- Decreased pO_2
- Decreased cooperation
- Apprehension
- Decreased SaO_2
- Increased use of accessory muscles

Related Factors

Respiratory muscle fatigue
Metabolic factors

* *Formerly "Inability to Sustain Spontaneous Ventilation"*

DYSFUNCTIONAL VENTILATORY WEANING RESPONSE
(1992)

Definition *Inability to adjust to lowered levels of mechanical ventilator support that interrupts and prolongs the weaning process*

Defining Characteristics

Severe

- Deterioration in arterial blood gases from current baseline
- Respiratory rate increases significantly from baseline
- Increase from baseline blood pressure (20 mm Hg)
- Agitation
- Increase from baseline heart rate (20 beats/min)
- Paradoxical abdominal breathing
- Adventitious breath sounds, audible airway secretions
- Cyanosis
- Decreased level of consciousness
- Full respiratory accessory muscle use
- Shallow, gasping breaths
- Profuse diaphoresis
- Discoordinated breathing with the ventilator

Moderate

- Slight increase from baseline blood pressure (<20 mm Hg)
- Baseline increase in respiratory rate (<5 breaths/ min)
- Slight increase from baseline heart rate (<20 beats/ min)
- Pale, slight cyanosis
- Slight respiratory accessory muscle use
- Inability to respond to coaching
- Inability to cooperate
- Apprehension
- Color changes
- Decreased air entry on auscultation
- Diaphoresis
- Eye widening, wide-eyed look
- Hypervigilance to activities

continued

Dysfunctional Ventilatory Weaning Response, *continued*

Mild

- Warmth
- Restlessness
- Slight increase of respiratory rate from baseline
- Queries about possible machine malfunction
- Expressed feelings of increased need for oxygen
- Fatigue
- Increased concentration on breathing
- Breathing discomfort

Related Factors

Psychological

Patient perceived inefficacy about the ability to wean

Powerlessness

Anxiety: moderate, severe

Knowledge deficit of the weaning process, patient role

Hopelessness

Fear

Decreased motivation

Decreased self-esteem

Insufficient trust in the nurse

Situational

Uncontrolled episodic energy demands or problems

History of multiple unsuccessful weaning attempts

Adverse environment (e.g., noisy, active environment, negative events in the room, low nurse-patient ratio, extended nurse absence from bedside, unfamiliar nursing staff)

History of ventilator dependence >4 days to 1 week

Inappropriate pacing of diminished ventilator support

Inadequate social support

Physiological

Inadequate nutrition

Sleep pattern disturbance

Uncontrolled pain or discomfort

Ineffective airway clearance

V

RISK FOR OTHER-DIRECTED VIOLENCE*
(1980, 1996)

Definition *At risk for behaviors in which an individual demonstrates that he/she can be physically, emotionally, and/or sexually harmful to others*

Risk Factors

Body language: Rigid posture, clenching of fists and jaw, hyperactivity, pacing, breathlessness, threatening stances

History of violence against others (e.g., hitting someone, kicking someone, spitting at someone, scratching someone, throwing objects at someone, biting someone, attempted rape, rape, sexual molestation, urinating/defecating on a person)

History of threats of violence (e.g., verbal threats against property, verbal threats against person, social threats, cursing, threatening notes/letters, threatening gestures, sexual threats)

History of violent anti-social behavior (e.g., stealing, insistent borrowing, insistent demands for privileges, insistent interruption of meetings, refusal to eat, refusal to take medication, ignoring instructions)

History of violence, indirect (e.g., tearing off clothes, ripping objects off walls, writing on walls, urinating on floor, defecating on floor, stamping feet, temper tantrum, running in corridors, yelling, throwing objects, breaking a window, slamming doors, sexual advances)

continued

V

* *Formerly "Risk for Violence: Directed at Others"*

Risk for Other-Directed Violence, *continued*

Neurological impairment (e.g., positive EEG, CAT, MRI, neurological findings; head trauma; seizure disorders)

Cognitive impairment (e.g., learning disabilities, attention deficit disorder, decreased intellectual functioning)

History of childhood abuse

History of witnessing family violence

Cruelty to animals

Firesetting

Pre/perinatal complications/abnormalities

History of drug/alcohol abuse

Pathological intoxication

Psychotic symptomatology (e.g., auditory, visual, command hallucinations; paranoid delusions; loose, rambling, or illogical thought processes)

Motor vehicle offenses (e.g., frequent traffic violations, use of a motor vehicle to release anger)

Suicidal behavior

Impulsivity

Availability/possession of weapon(s)

RISK FOR SELF-DIRECTED VIOLENCE*
(1994)

Definition   *At risk for behaviors in which an individual demonstrates that he/she can be physically, emotionally and/or sexually harmful to self*

Risk Factors

Suicidal ideation (frequent, intense prolonged)

Suicidal plan (clear and specific lethality; method and availability of destructive means)

History of multiple suicide attempts

Behavioral clues (e.g., writing forlorn love notes, directing angry messages at a significant other who has rejected the person, giving away personal items, taking out a large life insurance policy)

Verbal clues (e.g., talking about death, "better off without me," asking questions about lethal dosages of drugs)

Emotional status (hopelessness, despair, increased anxiety, panic, anger, hostility)

Mental health (severe depression, psychosis, severe personality disorder, alcoholism or drug abuse

Physical health (hypochondriasis, chronic or terminal illness)

Employment (unemployed, recent job loss/failure)

Age 15 – 19

Age over 45

Marital status (single, widowed, divorced)

Occupation (executive, administrator/owner of business, professional, semiskilled worker)

Conflictual interpersonal relationships

Family background (chaotic or conflictual, history of suicide)

continued

* *Formerly "Risk for Violence: Self-Directed"*

Risk for Self-Directed Violence, *continued*

Sexual orientation
(bisexual [active],
homosexual [inactive])
Personal resources (poor
achievement, poor
insight, affect unavail-
able and poorly
controlled)

Social resources (poor
rapport, socially isolated,
unresponsive family)
People who engage in
autoerotic sexual acts

V

IMPAIRED WALKING
(1998)

Definition *Limitation of independent movement within the environment on foot*

Defining Characteristics

- Impaired ability to
  - Climb stairs
  - Walk required distances
  - Walk on an incline or decline
  - Walk on uneven surfaces
  - Navigate curbs

Related Factors

To be developed

Note. Suggested Functional Level Classification:
  0 = Completely independent
  1 = Requires use of equipment or device
  2 = Requires help from another person, for assistance, supervision, or teaching
  3 = Requires help from another person and equipment or device
  4 = Dependent, does not participate in activity

W

Wandering
(2000)

Definition *Meandering, aimless or repetitive locomotion that exposes the individual to harm; frequently incongruent with boundaries, limits, or obstacles*

Defining Characteristics

- Frequent or continuous movement from place to place, often revisiting the same destinations
- Persistent locomotion in search of "missing" or unattainable people or places
- Haphazard locomotion
- Locomotion into unauthorized or private spaces
- Locomotion resulting in unintended leaving of a premise
- Long periods of locomotion without an apparent destination
- Fretful locomotion or pacing

- Inability to locate significant landmarks in a familiar setting
- Locomotion that cannot be easily dissuaded or redirected
- Following behind or shadowing a caregiver's locomotion
- Trespassing
- Hyperactivity
- Scanning, seeking, or searching behaviors
- Periods of locomotion interspersed with periods of nonlocomotion (e.g., sitting, standing, sleeping)
- Getting lost

Related Factors

Cognitive impairment, specifically memory and recall deficits, disorientation, poor visuoconstructive (or visuospatial) ability, language (primarily expressive) defects

Cortical atrophy
Premorbid behavior (e.g., outgoing, sociable personality; premorbid dementia)
Separation from familiar people and places

Sedation

Emotional state, especially frustration, anxiety, boredom, or depression (agitation)

Over/understimulating social or physical environment

Physiological state or need (e.g., hunger/thirst, pain, urination, constipation)

Time of day

W

Part 2

TAXONOMY II

Organization of the NANDA nursing diagnoses has evolved from an alphabetical listing in the mid-1980s to a conceptual system that guide the classification of nursing diagnoses in a taxonomy. This part of the book focuses on recent history and the domains, classes, diagnostic concepts, and nursing diagnoses approved in 2000 as Taxonomy II. The multiaxial structure of the taxonomy is discussed and nomenclature and coding conversion tables are included to assist in the transition from Taxonomy I to Taxonomy II.

History of the Development of Taxonomy II

Following the biennial conference in April 1994, the Taxonomy Committee met to place newly submitted diagnoses into the Taxonomy I revised structure. The committee had considerable difficulty, however, categorizing some of these diagnoses. Given this difficulty and the expanding numbers of submissions at level 1.4 and higher, the committee felt a new taxonomic structure might be viable. This possibility gave rise to considerable discussion as to how this might be accomplished in a scholarly and replicable way.

To begin, the committee agreed to determine if there were categories that arose naturally from the data. Round One of a naturalistic Q sort was completed at the 1994 conference. Round Two was completed later and the analysis presented at the 1996 biennial conference. That Q sort yielded 21 categories, far too many to be useful or practical.

In 1998, the Taxonomy Committee forwarded to the NANDA Board of Directors four Q sorts using different frameworks #1, reported in 1996, was naturalistic; #2 used Jenny's (1994) framework; #3 used the NOC framework (Johnson & Maas, 1997); and #4 used Gordon's (1998) functional health patterns framework. No one of these was entirely satisfactory, although Gordon's was the best. With Gordon's permission, we modified her framework slightly to create #5, which was presented to the membership in April 1998. At that meeting we invited the members to sort the diagnoses according to the domains we had selected. By the end of the meeting 40 usable sets of data were available for analysis. During data collection, members of the Taxonomy Committee took careful notes of questions asked, confusion expressed by participants, and suggestions made for improvements.

Based on the analysis of the data and the field notes, additional modifications to the framework were made. One domain of the original framework was divided into two to reduce the number of classes and diagnoses falling within it. A separate domain was added for growth and development since the original framework did not contain that domain. Several other domains were renamed to better reflect the content of the diagnoses within them. The final taxonomic structure is much less like Gordon's original, but has reduced misclassification errors and redundancies to near zero. This is a much desired state in a taxonomic structure.

Finally, definitions were developed for all the domains and classes within the structure. The definition of each diagnosis was then compared to that of the class and the domain in which it was placed. Revisions and modifications in the diagnosis placements were made to ensure maximum match among domain, class, and diagnoses. Figure 2.1 depicts the organization of domains and classes in Taxonomy II. Table 2.1 shows Taxonomy II with its 13 domains, 106 classes, and 155 diagnoses.

Structure of Taxonomy II

Scientists, informaticists, and managers of databases are the primary users of actual taxonomic structures. Clinicians rarely need to use one except for referencing. Clinicians are primarily concerned with the actual diagnoses within the taxonomy. However, familiarity with how the diagnostic language is structured will aid the clinician who needs to find information quickly. Thus a brief explanation of how the taxonomy is designed will help you understand the diagnoses within it.

Taxonomy II was designed to be multiaxial in its form, thereby substantially improving the flexibility of the nomenclature and allowing for easy additions and modifications.

There are seven axes

Axis 1 The diagnostic concept

Axis 2 Time (acute to chronic, short-term, long-term)

Axis 3 Unit of care (individual, family, community, target group)

Axis 4 Age (fetus to elder)

Axis 5 Potentiality (actual, risk for, opportunity or potential for growth/enhancement)

Axis 6 Descriptor (limits or specifies the meaning of the diagnostic concept; see page 219)

Axis 7 Topology (parts/regions of the body)

Definitions of the Axes

An axis, for the purpose of the NANDA taxonomy, is operationally defined as a dimension of the human response that is considered in the diagnostic process.

The axes are represented in the named/coded nursing diagnosis through their values. In some cases they are named explicitly, e.g., *ineffective community coping* and *compromised family coping,* in which the unit of care (in this instance "community" and "family") is named. "Ineffective" and "compromised" are from the descriptor axis (Axis 6).

In other cases the axis is implicit, e.g., *activity intolerance,* in which the individual is the unit of care. In some instances a particular axis may not be pertinent to a particular diagnosis, and therefore is not a part of the nursing diagnosis label or code. For example, the time axis with its four values may not be relevant to each diagnostic situation.

Axis 1 The Diagnostic Concept

The diagnostic concept is defined as the principal element or the fundamental and essential part, the root, of the diagnostic statement. The diagnostic concept may consist of one or more nouns. When more than one noun is used (e.g., *activity intolerance*), each one contributes to a unique meaning as if the two were a single noun; the meaning is different from the nouns stated separately. In some cases an adjective

Figure 2.1 Taxonomy II Domains and Classes

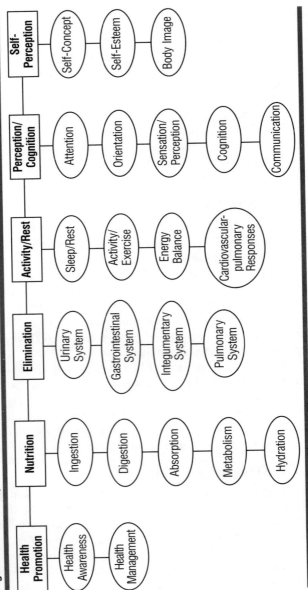

continued

Figure 2.1 *continued*

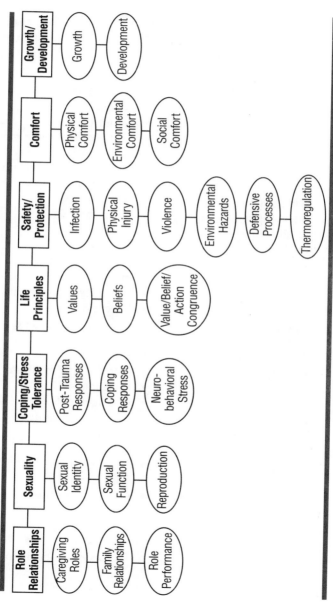

(e.g., spiritual) may be used with a noun (e.g., distress) to denote the diagnostic concept *spiritual distress*. The diagnostic concepts in Taxonomy II are:

- Activity intolerance
- Adjustment
- Airway clearance
- Anxiety
- Aspiration
- Attachment
- Autonomic dysreflexia
- Bed mobility
- Body image
- Body temperature
- Breastfeeding
- Breathing pattern
- Cardiac output
- Caregiver role strain
- Confusion
- Constipation
- Coping
- Death anxiety
- Decisional conflict
- Denial
- Dentition
- Development
- Diarrhea
- Disuse syndrome
- Diversional activity
- Elimination
- Energy field
- Environmental interpretation
- Failure to thrive
- Falls
- Family processes
- Fatigue
- Fear
- Fluid volume
- Gas exchange
- Grieving
- Growth
- Growth and development
- Health maintenance
- Health-seeking behaviors
- Home maintenance
- Hopelessness
- Hyperthermia
- Hypothermia
- Incontinence
- Identity disturbance
- Infant behavior
- Infant feeding pattern
- Infection
- Intracranial adaptive capacity
- Knowledge
- Latex allergy response
- Loneliness
- Management of therapeutic regimen
- Memory
- Nausea
- Noncompliance
- Nutrition
- Oral mucous membrane
- Pain
- Parenting
- Perfusion
- Perioperative-positioning injury
- Physical mobility

- Poisoning
- Post-trauma
- Powerlessness
- Protection
- Rape-trauma syndrome
- Relocation stress
- Role conflict
- Role performance
- Self-care
- Self-esteem
- Self-mutilation
- Sensory perception
- Sexual dysfunction
- Sexuality patterns
- Skin integrity
- Sleep deprivation
- Sleep pattern
- Social interaction
- Social isolation
- Sorrow
- Spiritual distress
- Spiritual well-being
- Spontaneous ventilation
- Suffocation
- Suicide
- Surgical recovery
- Swallowing
- Thermoregulation
- Thought processes
- Tissue integrity
- Transfer
- Trauma
- Unilateral neglect
- Urinary retention
- Ventilatory weaning response
- Verbal communication
- Violence
- Walking
- Wandering
- Wheelchair mobility

Axis 2 Time

Time is defined as the duration of a period or interval. Values in this axis are acute, chronic, intermittent, and continuous.

- *Acute:* Less than 6 months
- *Chronic:* More than 6 months
- *Intermittent:* Stopping or starting again at intervals, periodic, cyclic
- *Continuous:* Uninterrupted, going on without stop

Axis 3 The Unit of Care

The unit of care is defined as the distinct population for which a nursing diagnosis is determined. Values in Axis 3 are individual, family, group, and community

- *Individual:* A single human being distinct from others, a person.
- *Family:* Two or more people having continuous or sustained relationships, perceiving reciprocal obligations, sensing common meaning, and sharing certain obligations toward others; related by blood or choice.
- *Group:* Individuals gathered, classified, or acting together.
- *Community:* "'A group of people living in the same locale under the same government.' Examples include neighborhoods, cities, census tracts, and populations at risk." Craft-Rosenberg, 1999, p. 127)

When the unit of care is not explicitly stated, it becomes the individual by default.

Axis 4 Age

Age is defined as the length of time or interval during which an individual has existed. Values in Axis 4 are

- Fetus
- Neonate
- Infant
- Toddler
- Pre-school child
- School-age child

- Adolescent
- Young adult
- Middle-age adult
- Young old adult
- Middle old adult
- Old old adult

Axis 5 Health status

Health status is defined as the position or rank on the health continuum. Values in Axis 5 are wellness, risk, or actual:

- *Wellness:* The quality or state of being healthy especially as a result of deliberate effort.
- *Risk:* Vulnerability, especially as a result of exposure to factors that increase the chance of injury or loss.
- *Actual:* Existing in fact or reality, existing at the present time.

Axis 6 Descriptor

A descriptor or modifier is defined as a judgment that limits or specifies the meaning of a nursing diagnosis. Values in Axis 6 are:

- *Ability:* Capacity to do or act
- *Anticipatory:* To realize beforehand, foresee
- *Balance:* State of equilibrium
- *Compromised:* To make vulnerable to threat
- *Decreased:* Lessened; lesser in size, amount or degree
- *Deficient:* Inadequate in amount, quality or degree; not sufficient; incomplete
- *Delayed:* To postpone, impede, and retard
- *Depleted:* Emptied wholly or in part, exhausted of
- *Disproportionate:* Not consistent with a standard
- *Disabling:* To make unable or unfit, to incapacitate
- *Disorganized:* To destroy the systematic arrangement
- *Disturbed:* Agitated or interrupted, interfered with
- *Dysfunctional:* Abnormal, incomplete functioning
- *Effective:* Producing the intended or expected effect
- *Excessive:* Characterized by an amount or quantity that is greater than necessary, desirable, or useful
- *Functional:* Normal complete functioning
- *Imbalanced:* State of disequilibrium
- *Impaired:* Made worse, weakened, damaged, reduced, deteriorated
- *Inability:* Incapacity to do or act
- *Increased:* Greater in size, amount or degree
- *Ineffective:* Not producing the desired effect
- *Interrupted:* To break the continuity or uniformity
- *Organized:* To form as into a systematic arrangement
- *Perceived:* To become aware of by means of the senses; assignment of meaning
- *Readiness for enhanced* (for use with wellness diagnoses): To make greater, to increase in quality, to attain the more desired

Axis 7 Topology

The topology consists of parts/regions of the body—all tissues, organs, anatomical sites or structures. Values in Axis 7 are:

- Auditory
- Bowel
- Cardiopulmonary
- Cerebral
- Gastrointestinal
- Gustatory
- Intracranial
- Urinary
- Mucous membranes
- Oral
- Olfactory
- Peripheral neurovascular
- Peripheral vascular
- Renal
- Skin
- Tactile
- Visual

Because it is a multiaxial framework, you will notice that the descriptors (e.g., decreased, impaired) now appear on an axis separate from the diagnostic concepts. As the taxonomy develops, you may choose the diagnostic concept/human response that explains the situation with the individual client/patient; you may also choose the descriptor from those available on the descriptor axis. For example, if the human response of concern is parenting, you have a choice on the descriptor axis of *impaired* or *readiness for enhanced.* In addition, you have five other axes from which to choose appropriate items. For the parenting diagnosis, you might choose *individual* from the unit of care axis, *adolescent* from the age axis, and *risk for* from the health status axis to arrive at the diagnosis of *risk for impaired parenting, individual, adolescent.*

Some words of caution as well as encouragement: Using a multiaxial structure allows many diagnoses to be constructed that have no defining characteristics and may even be nonsense (such as "impaired activities of daily living, fetus"). We urge you to use only those diagnoses that are approved for testing and thus have defining characteristics.

(text continues on p. 232)

Table 2.1 Taxonomy II: Domains, Classes, Diagnostic Concepts, and Diagnoses

Domain 1 Health Promotion

The awareness of well-being or normality of function and the strategies used to maintain control of and enhance that well-being or normality of function

Class 1 Health Awareness Recognition of normal function and well-being

Class 2 Health Management Identifying, controlling, performing, and integrating activities to maintain health and well-being

Diagnostic Concepts	Approved Diagnoses	
Therapeutic regimen management	*00082*	*Effective therapeutic regimen management*
	00078	*Ineffective therapeutic regimen management*
	00080	*Ineffective family therapeutic regimen management*
	00081	*Ineffective community therapeutic regimen management*
Health-seeking behaviors	*00084*	*Health-seeking behaviors (specify)*
Health maintenance	*00099*	*Ineffective health maintenance*
Home maintenance	*00098*	*Impaired home maintenance*

Domain 2 Nutrition

The activities of taking in, assimilating, and using nutrients for the purposes of tissue maintenance, tissue repair, and the production of energy

Class 1 Ingestion Taking food or nutrients into the body

Diagnostic Concepts	Approved Diagnoses	
Infant feeding pattern	*00107*	*Ineffective infant feeding pattern*
Swallowing	*00103*	*Impaired swallowing*
Nutrition	*00002*	*Imbalanced nutrition: Less than body requirements*

continued

Table 2.1 *continued*

Diagnostic Concepts	Approved Diagnoses	
Nutrition	*00001*	*Imbalanced nutrition: More than body requirements*
	00003	*Risk for imbalanced nutrition: More than body requirements*

Class 2 Digestion The physical and chemical activities that convert foodstuffs into substances suitable for absorption and assimilation

Class 3 Absorption The act of taking up nutrients through body tissues

Class 4 Metabolism The chemical and physical processes occurring in living organisms and cells for the development and use of protoplasm, production of waste and energy, with the release of energy for all vital processes

Class 5 Hydration The taking in and absorption of fluids and electrolytes

Diagnostic Concepts	Approved Diagnoses	
Fluid volume	*00027*	*Deficient fluid volume*
	00028	*Risk for deficient fluid volume*
	00026	*Excess fluid volume*
	00025	*Risk for fluid volume imbalance*

Domain 3 Elimination
Secretion and excretion of waste products from the body

Class 1 Urinary System The process of secretion and excretion of urine

Diagnostic Concepts	Approved Diagnoses	
Urinary elimination	*00016*	*Impaired urinary elimination*
Urinary retention	*00023*	*Urinary retention*
Urinary incontinence	*00021*	*Total urinary incontinence*
	00020	*Functional urinary incontinence*
	00017	*Stress urinary incontinence*
	00019	*Urge urinary incontinence*
	00018	*Reflex urinary incontinence*
	00022	*Risk for urge urinary incontinence*

Class 2 *Gastrointestinal System* Excretion and expulsion of waste products from the bowel

Diagnostic Concepts	Approved Diagnoses	
Bowel incontinence	*00014*	*Bowel incontinence*
Diarrhea	*00013*	*Diarrhea*
Constipation	*00011*	*Constipation*
	00015	*Risk for constipation*
	00012	*Perceived constipation*

Class 3 *Integumentary System*
Process of secretion and excretion through the skin

Class 4 *Pulmonary System* Removal of byproducts of metabolic products, secretions, and foreign material from the lung or bronchi

Diagnostic Concepts	Approved Diagnoses	
Gas exchange	*00030*	*Impaired gas exchange*

Domain 4 Activity/Rest
The production, conservation, expenditure, or balance of energy resources

Class 1 *Sleep/Rest* Slumber, repose, ease, or inactivity

Diagnostic Concepts	Approved Diagnoses	
Sleep pattern	*00095*	*Disturbed sleep pattern*
	00096	*Sleep deprivation*

Class 2 *Activity/Exercise* Moving parts of the body (mobility), doing work, or performing actions often (but not always) against resistance

Diagnostic Concepts	Approved Diagnoses	
Disuse syndrome	*00040*	*Risk for disuse syndrome*
Mobility	*00085*	*Impaired physical mobility*
	00091	*Impaired bed mobility*
	00089	*Impaired wheelchair mobility*
Transfer ability	*00090*	*Impaired transfer ability*
Walking	*00088*	*Impaired walking*

continued

Table 2.1 *continued*

Diagnostic Concepts	Approved Diagnoses	
Diversional activity	*00097*	*Deficient diversional activity*
Wandering	*00154*	*Wandering*
Self-care deficit	*00109*	*Dressing/grooming deficit*
	00108	*Bathing/hygiene self-care deficit*
	00102	*Feeding self-care deficit*
	00110	*Toileting self-care deficit*
Surgical recovery	*00100*	*Delayed surgical recovery*

Class 3 Energy Balance A dynamic state of harmony between intake and expenditure of resources

Diagnostic Concepts	Approved Diagnoses	
Energy field	*00050*	*Disturbed energy field*
Fatigue	*00093*	*Fatigue*

Class 4 Cardiovascular/Pulmonary Responses
Cardiopulmonary mechanisms that support activity/rest

Diagnostic Concepts	Approved Diagnoses	
Cardiac output	*00029*	*Decreased cardiac output*
Spontaneous ventilation	*00033*	*Impaired spontaneous ventilation*
Breathing pattern	*00032*	*Ineffective breathing pattern*
Activity tolerance	*00092*	*Activity intolerance*
	00094	*Risk for activity intolerance*
Ventilatory weaning	*00034*	*Dysfunctional ventilatory weaning response*
Tissue perfusion	*00024*	*Ineffective tissue perfusion (specify type: renal, cerebral, cardiopulmonary, gastrointestinal, peripheral)*

Domain 5 Perception/Cognition
The human information processing system including attention, orientation, sensation, perception, cognition, and communication

Class 1 Attention Mental readiness to notice or observe

Diagnostic Concepts
Unilateral neglect

Approved Diagnoses
00123   Unilateral neglect

Class 2 Orientation Awareness of time, place, and person

Diagnostic Concepts
Environmental interpretation

Approved Diagnoses
00127   Impaired environmental interpretation syndrome

Class 3 Sensation/Perception Receiving information through the senses of touch, taste, smell, vision, hearing, and kinesthesia and the comprehension of sense data resulting in naming, associating, and/or pattern recognition

Diagnostic Concepts
Sensory perception

Approved Diagnoses
00122   Disturbed sensory perception (specify: visual, auditory, kinesthetic, gustatory, tactile, olfactory)

Class 4 Cognition Use of memory, learning, thinking, problem solving, abstraction, judgment, insight, intellectual capacity, calculation, and language

Diagnostic Concepts
Knowledge

Confusion

Memory

Thought processes

Approved Diagnoses
00126   Deficient knowledge (specify)

00128   Acute confusion
00129   Chronic confusion

00131   Impaired memory

00130   Disturbed thought processes

Class 5 Communication Sending and receiving verbal and nonverbal information

Diagnostic Concepts
Verbal communication

Approved Diagnoses
00051   Impaired verbal communication

Domain 6 Self-perception
Awareness about the self

Class 1 Self-Concept The perception(s) about the total self

continued

Table 2.1 *continued*

Diagnostic Concepts	Approved Diagnoses	
Identity	00121	Disturbed personal identity
	00125	Powerlessness
	00152	Risk for powerlessness
	00124	Hopelessness
Loneliness	00054	Risk for loneliness

Class 2   Self-esteem Assessment of one's own worth, capability, significance, and success

Diagnostic Concepts	Approved Diagnoses	
Self-esteem	00119	Chronic low self-esteem
	00120	Situational low self-esteem
	00153	Risk for situational low self-esteem

Class 3   Body Image A mental image of one's own body

Diagnostic Concepts	Approved Diagnoses	
Body image	00118	Disturbed body image

Domain 7 Role Relationships

The positive and negative connections or associations between persons or groups of persons and the means by which those connections are demonstrated

Class 1   Caregiving Roles Socially expected behavior patterns by persons providing care who are not health care professionals

Diagnostic Concepts	Approved Diagnoses	
Caregiver role strain	00061	Caregiver role strain
	00062	Risk for caregiver role strain
Parenting	00056	Impaired parenting
	00057	Risk for impaired parenting

Class 2   Family Relationships Associations of people who are biologically related or related by choice

Diagnostic Concepts	Approved Diagnoses	
Family processes	00060	Interrupted family processes

Diagnostic Concepts	Approved Diagnoses	
	00063	*Dysfunctional family processes: Alcoholism*
Attachment	*00058*	*Risk for impaired parent/infant/ child attachment*

Class 3 Role Performance Quality of functioning in socially expected behavior patterns

Diagnostic Concepts	Approved Diagnoses	
Breastfeeding	*00106*	*Effective breastfeeding*
	00104	*Ineffective breastfeeding*
	00105	*Interrupted breastfeeding*
Role performance	*00055*	*Ineffective role performance*
	00064	*Parental role conflict*
Social interaction	*00052*	*Impaired social interaction*

Domain 8 Sexuality
Sexual identity, sexual function, and reproduction

Class 1 Sexual Identity The state of being a specific person in regard to sexuality and/or gender

Class 2 Sexual Function The capacity or ability to participate in sexual activities

Diagnostic Concepts	Approved Diagnoses	
Sexual function	*00059*	*Sexual dysfunction*
Sexual patterns	*00065*	*Ineffective sexuality patterns*

Class 3 Reproduction Any process by which new individuals (people) are produced

Domain 9 Coping/Stress Tolerance
Contending with life events/life processes

Class 1 Post-Trauma Responses Reactions occurring after physical or psychological trauma

Diagnostic Concepts	Approved Diagnoses	
Relocation stress	*00114*	*Relocation stress syndrome*

continued

Table 2.1 *continued*

Diagnostic Concepts	Approved Diagnoses	
Relocation stress	*00149*	*Risk for relocation stress syndrome*
Rape-trauma	*00142*	*Rape-trauma syndrome*
	00144	*Rape-trauma syndrome: Silent reaction*
	00143	*Rape-trauma syndrome: Compound reaction*
Post-trauma response	*00141*	*Post-trauma syndrome*
	00145	*Risk for post-trauma syndrome*

Class 2 Coping Responses The process of managing environmental stress

Diagnostic Concepts	Approved Diagnoses	
Fear	*00148*	*Fear*
Anxiety	*00146*	*Anxiety*
	00147	*Death anxiety*
Sorrow	*00137*	*Chronic sorrow*
Denial	*00072*	*Ineffective denial*
	00136	*Anticipatory grieving*
	00135	*Dysfunctional grieving*
Adjustment	*00070*	*Impaired adjustment*
Coping	*00069*	*Ineffective coping*
	00073	*Disabled family coping*
	00074	*Compromised family coping*
	00071	*Defensive coping*
	00077	*Ineffective community coping*
	00075	*Readiness for enhanced family coping*
	00076	*Readiness for enhanced community coping*

Class 3 Neurobehavioral Stress Behavioral responses reflecting nerve and brain function

Diagnostic Concepts	Approved Diagnoses	
Dysreflexia	*00009*	*Autonomic dysreflexia*
	00010	*Risk for autonomic dysreflexia*
Infant behavior	*00116*	*Disorganized infant behavior*
	00115	*Risk for disorganized infant behavior*
	00117	*Readiness for enhanced organized infant behavior*
Adaptive capacity	*00049*	*Decreased intracranial adaptive capacity*

Domain 10 Life Principles

Principles underlying conduct, thought and behavior about acts, customs, or institutions viewed as being true or having intrinsic worth

Class 1 Values The identification and ranking of preferred modes of conduct or end states

Class 2 Beliefs Opinions, expectations, or judgments about acts, customs, or institutions viewed as being true or having intrinsic worth

Diagnostic Concepts	Approved Diagnoses	
Spiritual well-being	*00068*	*Readiness for enhanced spiritual well-being*

Class 3 Value/Belief/Action Congruence The correspondence or balance achieved between values, beliefs, and actions

Diagnostic Concepts	Approved Diagnoses	
Spiritual distress	*00066*	*Spiritual distress*
	00067	*Risk for spiritual distress*
Decisional conflict	*00083*	*Decisional conflict (specify)*
Noncompliance	*00079*	*Noncompliance (specify)*

Domain 11 Safety/Protection

Freedom from danger, physical injury or immune system damage, preservation from loss, and protection of safety and security

continued

Table 2.1 *continued*

Class 1 Infection Host responses following pathogenic invasion

Diagnostic Concepts	**Approved Diagnoses**	
Infection	00004	Risk for infection

Class 2 Physical Injury Bodily harm or hurt

Diagnostic Concepts	**Approved Diagnoses**	
Oral mucous membrane	00045	Impaired oral mucous membrane
Injury	00035	Risk for injury
	00087	Risk for perioperative positioning injury
	00155	Risk for falls
Trauma	00038	Risk for trauma
Skin integrity	00046	Impaired skin integrity
	00047	Risk for impaired skin integrity
Tissue integrity	00044	Impaired tissue integrity
Dentition	00048	Impaired dentition
Suffocation	00036	Risk for suffocation
Aspiration	00039	Risk for aspiration
Airway clearance	00031	Ineffective airway clearance
Neurovascular function	00086	Risk for peripheral neurovascular dysfunction
Protection	00043	Ineffective protection

Class 3 Violence The exertion of excessive force or power so as to cause injury or abuse

Diagnostic Concepts	**Approved Diagnoses**	
Self-mutilation	00139	Risk for self-mutilation
	00151	Self-mutilation
Violence	00138	Risk for other-directed violence
	00140	Risk for self-directed violence
	00150	Risk for suicide

Class 4 **Environmental Hazards** Sources of danger in the surroundings

Diagnostic Concepts
Poisoning

Approved Diagnoses
00037   Risk for poisoning

Class 5 **Defensive Processes** The processes by which the self protects itself from the nonself

Diagnostic Concepts
Latex allergy response

Approved Diagnoses
00041   Latex allergy response
00042   Risk for latex allergy response

Class 6 **Thermoregulation** The physiologic process of regulating heat and energy within the body for purposes of protecting the organism

Diagnostic Concepts
Body temperature

Thermoregulation

Approved Diagnoses
00005   Risk for imbalanced body temperature

00008   Ineffective thermoregulation
00006   Hypothermia
00007   Hyperthermia

Domain 12 Comfort
Sense of mental, physical, or social well-being or ease

Class 1 **Physical Comfort** Sense of well-being or ease

Diagnostic Concepts
Pain

Nausea

Approved Diagnoses
00132   Acute pain
00133   Chronic pain

00134   Nausea

Class 2 **Environmental Comfort** Sense of well-being or ease in/with one's environment

Class 3 **Social Comfort** Sense of well-being or ease with one's social situations

Diagnostic Concepts
Social isolation

Approved Diagnoses
00053   Social isolation

continued

Table 2.1 *continued*

Domain 13 Growth/Development
Age-appropriate increases in physical dimensions, organ systems, and/or attainment of developmental milestones

Class 1 Growth Increases in physical dimensions or maturity of organ systems

Diagnostic Concepts	Approved Diagnoses	
Growth	00113	*Risk for disproportionate growth*
Failure to thrive	00101	*Adult failure to thrive*

Class 2 Development Attainment, lack of attainment, or loss of developmental milestones

Diagnostic Concepts	Approved Diagnoses	
Development	00111	*Delayed growth and development*
	00112	*Risk for delayed development*

Further Development of Taxonomy II Nursing Diagnoses

A multiaxial framework allows clinicians to see where there are gaps and/or potentially useful new diagnoses. If you construct a new diagnosis or a set of diagnoses that is useful to your practice, please submit it to NANDA so others can share in the benefit. Submission guidelines are on page 241. Submission forms can be found on the NANDA Web site: www.NANDA.org. The Diagnostic Review Committee will be glad to help you with your submission.

Code Conversion: Taxonomy I to Taxonomy II

Taxonomy II has a code structure that is compliant with recommendations from the National Library of Medicine (NLM) concerning healthcare terminology codes. The NLM recommends that codes not contain information on location, as did the Taxonomy I code structure. The original structure gave information about the location of a diagnosis within a classification—e.g., all diagnoses in the Exchanging pattern began with a 1.

The Taxonomy II code structure is a 32-bit integer (if your database uses another notation, it is a 5-digit code). This structure provides for the evolution of the classification structure as a result of knowledge development without having to change the codes of the diagnoses.

Table 2.2 shows the conversion from Taxonomy I codes to Taxonomy II codes, and provides codes for the new diagnoses.

Table 2.2 Code Conversion: Taxonomy I to Taxonomy II

Nursing Diagnosis	Taxonomy I Codes	Taxonomy II Codes
Exchanging	1	Retired
Imbalanced nutrition: More than body requirements	1.1.2.1	00001
Imbalanced nutrition: Less than body requirements	1.1.2.2	00002
Risk for imbalanced nutrition: More than body requirements	1.1.2.3	00003
Risk for infection	1.2.1.1	00004
Risk for imbalanced body temperature	1.2.2.1	00005
Hypothermia	1.2.2.2	00006
Hyperthermia	1.2.2.3	00007
Ineffective thermoregulation	1.2.2.4	00008
Autonomic dysreflexia	1.2.3.1	00009
Risk for autonomic dysreflexia	1.2.3.2	00010
Constipation	1.3.1.1	00011
Perceived constipation	1.3.1.1.1	00012
Diarrhea	1.3.1.2	00013
Bowel Incontinence	1.3.1.3	00014
Risk for constipation	1.3.1.4	00015
Impaired urinary elimination	1.3.2	00016
Stress urinary incontinence	1.3.2.1.1	00017
Reflex urinary incontinence	1.3.2.1.2	00018
Urge urinary incontinence	1.3.2.1.3	00019
Functional urinary incontinence	1.3.2.1.4	00020
Total urinary incontinence	1.3.2.1.5	00021
Risk for urge urinary incontinence	1.3.2.1.6	00022

continued

Table 2.2 *continued*

Nursing Diagnosis	Taxonomy I Codes	Taxonomy II Codes
Urinary retention	1.3.2.2	00023
Ineffective tissue perfusion (specify type: renal, cerebral, cardiopulmonary, gastrointestinal, peripheral)	1.4.1.1	00024
Risk for fluid volume imbalance	1.4.1.2	00025
Excess fluid volume	1.4.1.2.1	00026
Deficient fluid volume	1.4.1.2.2.1	00027
Risk for deficient fluid volume	1.4.1.2.2.2	00028
Decreased cardiac output	1.4.2.1	00029
Impaired gas exchange	1.5.1.1	00030
Ineffective airway clearance	1.5.1.2	00031
Ineffective breathing pattern	1.5.1.3	00032
Impaired spontaneous ventilation	1.5.1.3.1	00033
Dysfunctional ventilatory weaning response	1.5.1.3.2	00034
Risk for injury	1.6.1	00035
Risk for suffocation	1.6.1.1	00036
Risk for poisoning	1.6.1.2	00037
Risk for trauma	1.6.1.3	00038
Risk for aspiration	1.6.1.4	00039
Risk for disuse syndrome	1.6.1.5	00040
Latex allergy response	1.6.1.6	00041
Risk for latex allergy response	1.6.1.7	00042
Ineffective protection	1.6.2	00043
Impaired tissue integrity	1.6.2.1	00044
Impaired oral mucous membrane	1.6.2.1.1	00045
Impaired skin integrity	1.6.2.1.2.1	00046
Risk for impaired skin integrity	1.6.2.1.2.2	00047
Impaired dentition	1.6.2.1.2.3	00048
Decreased intracranial adaptive capacity	1.7.1	00049
Disturbed energy field	1.8	00050
Communicating	2	Retired
Impaired verbal communication	2.1.1.1	00051
Relating	3	Retired
Impaired social interaction	3.1.1	00052
Social isolation	3.1.2	00053

Nursing Diagnosis	Taxonomy I Codes	Taxonomy II Codes
Risk for loneliness	3.1.3	00054
Ineffective role performance	3.2.1	00055
Deficient parenting	3.2.1.1.1	00056
Risk for deficient parenting	3.2.1.1.2	00057
Risk for impaired parent/infant/child attachment	3.2.1.1.2.1	00058
Sexual dysfunction	3.2.1.2.1	00059
Interrupted family processes	3.2.2	00060
Caregiver role strain	3.2.2.1	00061
Risk for caregiver role strain	3.2.2.2	00062
Dysfunctional family processes: Alcoholism	3.2.2.3.1	00063
Parental role conflict	3.2.3.1	00064
Ineffective sexuality patterns	3.3	00065
Valuing	4	Retired
Spiritual distress	4.1.1	00066
Risk of spiritual distress	4.1.2	00067
Readiness for enhanced spiritual well-being	4.2	00068
Choosing	5	Retired
Ineffective coping	5.1.1.1	00069
Impaired adjustment	5.1.1.1.1	00070
Defensive coping	5.1.1.1.2	00071
Ineffective denial	5.1.1.1.3	00072
Disabled family coping	5.1.2.1.1	00073
Compromised family coping	5.1.2.1.2	00074
Readiness for enhanced family coping	5.1.2.2	00075
Readiness for enhanced community coping	5.1.3.1	00076
Ineffective community coping	5.1.3.2	00077
Ineffective therapeutic regimen management	5.2.1	00078
Noncompliance (specify)	5.2.1.1	00079
Ineffective family therapeutic regimen management	5.2.2	00080
Ineffective community therapeutic regimen management	5.2.3	00081
Effective therapeutic regimen management	5.2.4	00082
Decisional conflict (specify)	5.3.1.1	00083

continued

Table 2.2 *continued*

Nursing Diagnosis	Taxonomy I Codes	Taxonomy II Codes
Health-seeking behaviors (specify)	5.4	00084
Moving	6	Retired
Impaired physical mobility	6.1.1.1	00085
Risk for peripheral neurovascular dysfunction	6.1.1.1.1	00086
Risk for perioperative-positioning injury	6.1.1.1.2	00087
Impaired walking	6.1.1.1.3	00088
Impaired wheelchair mobility	6.1.1.1.4	00089
Impaired transfer ability	6.1.1.1.5	00090
Impaired bed mobility	6.1.1.1.6	00091
Activity intolerance	6.1.1.2	00092
Fatigue	6.1.1.2.1	00093
Risk for activity intolerance	6.1.1.3	00094
Disturbed sleep pattern	6.2.1	00095
Sleep deprivation	6.2.1.1	00096
Deficient diversional activity	6.3.1.1	00097
Impaired home maintenance	6.4.1.1	00098
Ineffective health maintenance	6.4.2	00099
Delayed surgical recovery	6.4.2.1	00100
Adult failure to thrive	6.4.2.2	00101
Feeding self-care deficit	6.5.1	00102
Impaired swallowing	6.5.1.1	00103
Ineffective breastfeeding	6.5.1.2	00104
Interrupted breastfeeding	6.5.1.2.1	00105
Effective breastfeeding	6.5.1.3	00106
Ineffective infant feeding pattern	6.5.1.4	00107
Bathing/hygiene self-care deficit	6.5.2	00108
Dressing/grooming self-care deficit	6.5.3	00109
Toileting self-care deficit	6.5.4	00110
Delayed growth and development	6.6	00111
Risk for delayed development	6.6.1	00112
Risk for disproportionate growth	6.6.2	00113
Relocation stress syndrome	6.7	00114
Risk for disorganized infant behavior	6.8.1	00115
Disorganized infant behavior	6.8.2	00116

Nursing Diagnosis	Taxonomy I Codes	Taxonomy II Codes
Readiness for enhanced organized infant behavior	6.8.3	00117
Perceiving	7	Retired
Disturbed body image	7.1.1	00118
Disturbed self-esteem	7.1.2	Retired
Chronic low self-esteem	7.1.2.1	00119
Situational low self-esteem	7.1.2.2	00120
Disturbed personal identity	7.1.3	00121
Disturbed sensory perception (specify: visual, auditory, kinesthetic, gustatory, tactile, ol factory)	7.2	00122
Unilateral neglect	7.2.1.1	00123
Hopelessness	7.3.1	00124
Powerlessness	7.3.2	00125
Knowing	8	
Deficient knowledge (specify)	8.1.1	00126
Impaired environmental interpretation syndrome	8.2.1	00127
Acute confusion	8.2.2	00128
Chronic Confusion	8.2.3	00129
Disturbed thought processes	8.3	00130
Impaired memory	8.3.1	00131
Feeling	9	Retired
Acute pain	9.1.1	00132
Chronic pain	9.1.1.1	00133
Nausea	9.1.2	00134
Dysfunctional grieving	9.2.1.1	00135
Anticipatory grieving	9.2.1.2	00136
Chronic sorrow	9.2.1.3	00137
Risk for other-directed violence	9.2.2	00138
Risk for self-mutilation	9.2.2.1	00139
Risk for self-directed violence	9.2.2.2	00140
Post-trauma syndrome	9.2.3	00141
Rape-trauma syndrome	9.2.3.1	00142
Rape-trauma syndrome: Compound reaction	9.2.3.1.1	00143
Rape-trauma syndrome: Silent reaction	9.2.3.1.2	00144

continued

Table 2.2 *continued*

Nursing Diagnosis	Taxonomy I Codes	Taxonomy II Codes
Risk for post-trauma syndrome	9.2.4	00145
Anxiety	9.3.1	00146
Death anxiety	9.3.1.1	00147
Fear	9.3.2	00148
New Nursing Diagnoses, April 2000		
Risk for relocation stress syndrome		00149
Risk for suicide		00150
Self-mutilation		00151
Risk for powerlessness		00152
Risk for situational low self-esteem		00153
Wandering		00154
Risk for falls		00155

References

Braham, C.G., & the Random House Reference Staff (Eds.). (1998). *Random House Webster's dictionary* (3rd ed.). New York: Ballantine Books.

Craft-Rosenberg, M. (1999). Notes on NDEC: Diagnoses for community nursing. *Nursing Diagnosis, 10,* 127–129.

Gordon, M. (1998). *Manual of nursing diagnosis.* St. Louis: Mosby.

Jenny, J. (1994). Advancing the science of nursing with nursing diagnosis. In M. Rantz & P. LeMone (Eds.), *Classification of nursing diagnoses: Proceedings of the eleventh conference* (pp. 73–81), Glendale, CA: CINAHL.

Johnson, M., & Maas, M. (1997). *Nursing outcomes classification (NOC).* St. Louis: Mosby.

NANDA. (1999). *NANDA nursing diagnoses: Definitions & classification 1999–2000.* Philadelphia: Author.

Part 3

NURSING DIAGNOSIS DEVELOPMENT

Diagnosis Submission Guidelines

New diagnoses and revisions of diagnoses submitted to NANDA undergo a systematic review to determine consistency with the established criteria for a nursing diagnosis. All submissions are subsequently staged according to evidence supporting either the level of development or validation. Further information on submission and the review process may be obtained by requesting a "Submission/Revision Packet" from NANDA, 1211 Locust St., Philadelphia, PA 19107; 800.647.9002; www.nanda.org

Diagnoses may be submitted at various levels of development (e.g., label and definition; label, definition, defining characteristics, related factors). Any submission beyond that of label and definition must include an integrative review of the literature and use the submission/review packet that is available from the NANDA office; additional research from related disciplines is also appropriate. Articles used for the submission are to be catalogued on a Literature Review Form (see submission/review packet).

A 3½" disk and a printed copy of all diagnoses are to be submitted in the format provided in the packet. The submitter is asked to compare his/her submission with all current related NANDA diagnoses (see example in submission/review packet).

On receipt, the diagnosis will be assigned to a primary reviewer from the Diagnosis Review Committee (DRC). This person will work with you as the DRC reviews your submission. Once the diagnosis is formally reviewed by DRC, it will be sent to nursing specialty group experts and the NANDA International Committee for comment. Recommendations will be shared with you. Diagnoses will then be discussed at forums at the next NANDA biennial conference in order to invite extended member input. Recommendations from the forums will be reviewed and the diagnoses forwarded to the NANDA Board of Directors. All diagnoses accepted at the 2.1 level of development are then included in NANDA's publication, *Nursing Diagnoses: Definitions & Classification.*

Diagnosis Staging Criteria

2.0 Accepted for Clinical Development (Authentication/ Substantiation)

2.1 Label, Definition, Defining Characteristics or Risk Factors, References, and Literature Review

At Stage 2.1, the label is forwarded to the Taxonomy Committee for classification. A narrative review of relevant literature is required to demonstrate the existence of a substantive body of knowledge underlying the diagnosis. The literature review is consistent with the label and definition. Literature should include discussion and support of the defining characteristics or risk factors (for risk diagnoses) and related factors (for actual diagnoses).

2.2 Case Study

The criteria in 2.1 are met. The narrative includes description of an actual case that exhibits the nursing diagnosis and includes defining characteristics or risk factors. Related factors, interventions, and outcomes are optional.

2.3 Clinical Case Studies

The criteria in 2.1 and 2.2 are met. The narrative includes the description of a series of at least 10 cases that exhibit the diagnosis and include defining characteristics or risk factors, related factors, interventions, and outcomes.

2.4 Consensus Studies Related to Diagnosis Using Nurse Experts

The above criteria are met. Studies include opinionnaire, Delphi, and similar studies of diagnostic components (e.g., diagnostic content validity) in which nurses are the subjects.

3.0 Clinically Supported (Validation and Testing)

3.1 Clinical Studies Related to Diagnosis, But Not Generalizeable to the Population

The criteria in 2.3 are met. The narrative includes a description of studies related to the diagnosis, which includes defining characteristics or risk factors, and related factors. Studies may be qualitative in nature, or quantitative studies using nonrandom samples in which patients are the subjects.

3.2 Well-Designed Clinical Studies With Small Sample Sizes

The criteria in 2.3 are met. The narrative includes a description of studies related to the diagnosis, which includes defining characteristics or risk factors, and related factors. Random sampling is used in these studies, but sample size is limited.

3.3 Well-Designed Clinical Studies With Random Sample of Sufficient Size to Allow for Generalizeablility to the Overall Population

The criteria in 2.3 are met. The narrative includes a description of studies related to the diagnosis, which includes defining characteristics or risk factors, and related factors. Random sampling is used in these studies; sample size is sufficient to allow for generalizeability of results to the overall population.

T. Heather Herdman, PhD, RN
Chair, Diagnosis Review Committee

Glossary of Terms Used by NANDA

Nursing Diagnoses

Nursing diagnosis A clinical judgment about individual, family, or community responses to actual or potential health problems/life processes. A nursing diagnosis provides the basis for selection of nursing interventions to achieve outcomes for which the nurse is accountable (approved at the 9th conference, 1990).

Actual nursing diagnosis Describes human responses to health conditions/life processes that exist in an individual, family, or community. It is supported by defining characteristics (manifestations, signs and symptoms) that cluster in patterns of related cues or inferences.

Risk nursing diagnosis Describes human responses to health conditions/life processes that may develop in a vulnerable individual, family, or community. It is supported by risk factors that contribute to increased vulnerability.

Wellness nursing diagnosis Describes human responses to levels of wellness in an individual, family, or community that have a readiness for enhancement.

Components of a Diagnosis

Label Provides a name for a diagnosis. It is a concise term or phrase that represents a pattern of related cues. It may include modifiers.

Definition Provides a clear, precise description; delineates its meaning; and helps differentiate it from similar diagnoses.

Defining characteristics Observable cues/inferences that cluster as manifestations of an actual or wellness nursing diagnosis.

Risk factors Environmental factors and physiological, psychological, genetic, or chemical elements that increase the vulnerability of an individual, family, or community to an unhealthful event.

Related factors Factors that appear to show some type of patterned relationship with the nursing diagnosis. Such factors may be described as antecedent to, associated with, related to, contributing to, or abetting.

Definitions for Classification of Nursing Diagnoses

Classification Systematic arrangement of related phenomena in groups or classes based on characteristics that objects have in common

Level of abstraction Describes the concreteness/abstractness of a concept. (a) Very abstract concepts are theoretical, may not be directly measurable, defined by concrete concepts, inclusive of concrete concepts, disassociated from any specific instance, independent of time and space, have more general descriptors, may not be clinically useful for planning treatment. (b) Concrete concepts are observable and measurable, limited by time and space, constitute a specific category, more exclusive, name a real thing or class of things, restricted by nature, may be clinically useful for planning treatment.

Nomenclature A system of designations (terms) elaborated according to pre-established rules (American Nurses Association)

Taxonomy Classification according to presumed natural relationships among types and their subtypes (American Nurses Association [ANA], 1999).

Reference

American Nurses Association. (1999). *ANA CNP II recognition criteria and definitions*. Washington, DC: Author.

NANDA Guidelines for Copyright Permission

The materials presented in this book are copyrighted and all copyright laws apply. Situations requiring approvals and/or copyright fees are listed below:

1. An author or publishing house requests use of the entire nursing diagnosis taxonomy in a textbook or other nursing manual to be sold.
2, An author or publishing house requests use of only the list of nursing diagnoses with no definitions or defining characteristics.
3. An author or company requests use of the nursing diagnosis taxonomy in audio-visual material.
4. A software developer or computer-based patient record vendor requests use of the nursing diagnosis taxonomy in a program.
5. A nursing school, researcher, professional organization, or health care organization requests use of the nursing diagnosis taxonomy in a program.

Send all reproduction permission requests to NANDA, 1211 Locust St., Philadelphia, PA 19107, USA; phone: 800.647.9002/215.545.7222; fax: 215.545.8107; e-mail: nanda@rmpinc.com.

NANDA Board of Directors

President: Kay Avant, PhD, RN, FAAN
President-Elect: Mary Ann Lavin, ScD, RN, CS, ANP, FAAN
Secretary: Meridean Maas, PhD, RN, FAAN
Treasurer: Sheila Sparks, DNSc, RN, CS
Directors:
　Marjory Gordon, PhD, RN, FAAN
　Anne Perry, EdD, RN
　Judith Warren, PhD, RN, FAAN
　Georgia Griffith Whitley, EdD, RN

NANDA Diagnosis Review Committee

T. Heather Herdman, PhD, RN, *Chair*
Lynda Juall Carpenito, MSN, RN, CRNP
Jean O'Neil, EdD, RN
Leann Scroggins, MSN, RN
Georgia Griffith Whitley, EdD, RN, *Board Liaison*

NANDA Taxonomy Committee

Lois Hoskins, PhD, RN, FAAN, *Chair*
Martha Craft-Rosenberg, PhD, RN, FAAN
Barbara Vassallo, EdD, RN, CS, ANPC
Ann Woodtli, PhD, RN, FAAN
Judith Warren, PhD, RN, FAAN, *Board Liaison*

Nursing Diagnosis Extension and Classification (NDEC) Research Team

Principal Investigators
　Martha Craft-Rosenberg, PhD, RN, FAAN,
　Connie Delaney, PhD, RN, FAAN
　Janice Denehy, PhD, RN

NDEC Investigators
　JoAnn Chapman, MPH, BS, RN, PCA
　Dame June Clark, DBE, PhD, RN, RHV, FRNC
　Mary Clarke, MA, RN
　Judith A. Collins, MA, ARNP, CNS
　Carolyn M. Crowell, MN, RN
　Mary Patricia Donahue, PhD, RN, FAAN
　Orpha Glick, PhD, RN
　Cyd Q. Grafft, MS, RN, ARNP
　Joseph E. Grieiner, MSN, RN

Jone Johnson, MA, RN
Kathleen Hanson, PhD, RN
Meridean Maas, PhD, RN, FAAN
Leslie Marshall, PhD, RN
Sandra Powell, PhD, RN
Colleen Prophet, MA, RN
Jean Reese, PhD, RN
Lavonne Ruther, MA, RN
Deborah Jensen Schoenfelder, PhD, RN
Lucina Sheehy, MS, RN
Janet Specht, PhD, RN, FAAN

Members of Diagnosis Work Groups

Denise Antle, BSN, RN, CCRN
Lisa Burkhart, MPH, RN
Veronica Brighton, MA, RN, ARNP, CS
Amy Coenen, PhD, RN, CS
Regina Murphy, MSN, RN, ARNP
Lisa Skemp Kelley, PhD(C), RN, MA,
Lois Holz, BSN, RN
Rebecca Jacobs, MA, RN, C
Charmaine Kleiber, MS, DNC
Darcy Koehn, MA, RN
Janice Kruse, BSN, RN, C
Karen LeMaster, MA, RN, CAN, CCRN
Anne Lewis, MA, RN
Ann Marie McCarthy, PhD, RN, PNP
Karen Nelson, BSN, RN
Linda A. Petersen, BSN, RNC, Master's candidate
Thomas J. Martz, RN, MSN
Lou Ann Montgomery, MA, RN, CCNS, CCRN
Carralee Sueppel, MS, RN
Joanne Tigges, MA, RN
Janet Williams, PhD, RN, PNP, FAAN
James Waterman, MS, RN

Chairs, NDEC Satellite Groups

Donna L. Algase, PhD
Mary Jane Oakland, PhD, RD, LD, FADA

An Invitation to Join NANDA

Purpose of NANDA

The purpose of NANDA is to develop, refine, and promote a taxonomy of nursing diagnostic terminology of general use to the professional nurse.

Functions of the Organization

1. Provide a structure for formalizing the language describing the phenomena of concern to nursing.
2. Provide a system for developing and refining nursing diagnoses.
3. Facilitate nursing diagnosis research.
4. Publish proceedings of the biennial conferences.
5. Publish a quarterly journal.
6. Provide support, communication, and resources through conferences, publications, and networking.

Membership Requirements

Membership is open to all registered nurses with a current RN license. Associate membership is extended to nonregistered nurses and students who share an interest in the purpose of the association.

Organizational Background

NANDA was formed in 1982, replacing the National Conference Group established in 1973. NANDA has approved 155 diagnoses for clinical testing and refinement.

A dynamic process of diagnosis review and taxonomy development continues toward identifying and classifying nursing phenomena. NANDA diagnoses are included in the Unified Medical Language System of the National Library of Medicine, and NANDA is working with the American Nurses Association in developing a Unified Nursing Language System. NANDA is also cooperating with the International Council of Nurses to develop an International Classification of Nursing Practice.

Benefits of Membership

1. Subscription to *Nursing Diagnosis: The International Journal of Nursing Language and Classification.*
2. Reduced registration fee at the biennial conference.
3. Participation in decisions about new and revised diagnoses.
4. State-of-the-art information on development of nursing language systems.
5. Reduced rate on in-house publications.
6. Information resource for networking and research data.

Additional Materials Available

NANDA publishes its taxonomy in *NANDA Nursing Diagnoses: Definitions & Classification.* A new edition is printed after each biennial conference. This book contains the only list of diagnoses approved by NANDA far distribution.

To order or obtain information on NANDA publications, including the conference proceedings, contact the NANDA office:

1211 Locust St.
Philadelphia, PA 19107
Phone: 800.647.9002
Fax: 215.545.8107
E-mail: nanda@rmpinc.com
Web: www.nanda.org

For conference information, contact the NANDA office.

NANDA MEMBERSHIP APPLICATION

Last Name:_____First:_____ MI:____

Home Address: _____

City/State/Zip/Country: _____

Home telephone number: _____

Fax number: _____ E-mail: _____

Place of Employment: _____

Position or Title: _____

Business address: _____

City/State/Zip/Country: _____

Business telephone number: _____

Fax number: _____ E-mail: _____

Current RN license number: _____

State/province/country: _____

Demographic data (circle one in each category):

Initial nursing education: Diploma, Associate degree, Baccalaureate degree, Other highest degree held: BS, BSN, MS, MSN, PhD, DNSc, EdD; Other primary function: Administrator, Manager, Clinician, Staff Nurse, Consultant, Educator, Researcher Clinical Nurse Specialist, Nurse Practitioner, Other (Specify)

Area of specialization: Community Health, Maternal/Newborn, Parent/Child, Medical/Surgical, Nursing of Children, Critical Care, Psychiatry/Mental Health, Gerontology, Long-Term Care, Health Promotion, Nursing Administration, Rehabilitation, Perioperative Nursing, Ambulatory Care, Nursing Informatics

Are you a member of the ANA? Yes____ No____

Membership Fee

Regular membership: $100.00[a]   Retired RN membership: $65.00[a]

Student membership: $29.00   Associate Membership: $100.00[a]

Indicate Method of Payment: Checks[b] or money orders should be made payable to NANDA.

Check___ Money Order ___ MasterCard___ VISA___

If using credit card complete:

Card No: _____

Exp. Date: _____ Signature: _____

Copy this application form and send it to:

NANDA, 1211 Locust St., Philadelphia, PA 19107; Fax 215.545.8107

[a]$29.00 is for a subscription to *Nursing Diagnosis: The International Journal of Nursing Language & Classification.*

[b]NANDA cannot accept checks in foreign currencies.

Index

Activity intolerance, 13
   Risk for, 14
Acute confusion, 47
Acute pain, 129
Adaptive capacity, Decreased
   intracranial, 112
Adjustment, Impaired, 15
Adult failure to thrive, 71
Airway clearance, ineffective,
   16
Alcoholism, Dysfunctional
   family processes, 75
Allergy response, Latex, 17
   Risk for, 18
Anticipatory grieving, 87
Anxiety, 19
   Death, 22
Aspiration, Risk for, 23
Attachment, Risk for
   impaired parent/
   infant/child, 24
Autonomic dysreflexia, 25
   Risk for, 26
Bathing/hygiene self-care
   deficit, 151
Bed mobility, Impaired, 116
Body image, Disturbed, 28
Body temperature, Risk for
   imbalanced, 30
Bowel incontinence, 31
Breastfeeding,
   Effective, 32
   Ineffective, 33
   Interrupted, 34
Breathing pattern, Ineffective,
   35
Cardiac output, Decreased, 36
Caregiver role strain, 38
   Risk for, 41

Chronic
   Confusion, 48
   Pain, 130
   Sorrow, 174
Communication, Impaired
   verbal, 43
Compromised family coping,
   58
Conflict
   Decisional, 45
   Parental role, 46
Confusion
   Acute, 47
   Chronic, 48
Constipation, 49
   Perceived, 51
   Risk for, 52
Coping,
   Defensive, 57
   Ineffective, 54
Coping, Community
   Ineffective, 55
   Readiness for enhanced, 56
Coping, Family
   Compromised, 58
   Disabled, 60
   Readiness for enhanced, 62
Death anxiety, 22
Decisional conflict, 45
Decreased cardiac output, 36
Denial, Ineffective, 63
Dentition, Impaired, 64
Development, Risk for
   delayed, 65
Diarrhea, 66
Disproportionate growth,
   Risk for, 90
Disturbed body image, 28
Disuse syndrome, Risk for, 67

Diversional activity, Deficient, 68

Dressing/grooming self-care deficit, 152

Dysreflexia, Autonomic, 25

Elimination, Impaired urinary, 196

Energy field, Disturbed, 69

Environmental interpretation syndrome, Impaired, 70

Excess fluid volume, 83

Failure to thrive, Adult, 71

Falls, Risk for, 73

Family processes
  Dysfunctional: Alcoholism, 75
  Interrupted, 78

Fatigue, 79

Fear, 80

Feeding self-care deficit, 153

Fluid volume
  Deficient, 82
  Excess, 83
  Risk for deficient, 84
  Risk for imbalanced, 85

Gas exchange, Impaired, 86

Grieving
  Anticipatory, 87
  Dysfunctional, 88

Growth and development, Delayed, 89

Growth, Risk for dispropor-tionate, 90

Health maintenance, Ineffective, 91

Health-seeking behaviors, 92

Home maintenance, Impaired, 93

Hopelessness, 94

Hyperthermia, 95

Hypothermia, 96

Identity, Disturbed personal, 97

Imbalanced fluid volume, Risk for, 85

Incontinence
  Bowel, 31
  Functional urinary, 98
  Reflex urinary, 99
  Stress urinary, 100
  Total urinary, 101
  Urge urinary, 102
  Urge urinary, Risk for, 103

Infant behavior
  Disorganized, 104
  Readiness for enhanced organized, 107
  Risk for disorganized, 106

Infant feeding pattern, Ineffective, 108

Infection, Risk for, 109

Injury
  Perioperative-positioning, Risk for, 111
  Risk for, 110

Intracranial adaptive capacity, Decreased, 112

Interrupted breastfeeding, 34

Knowledge, Deficient, 113

Latex allergy response, 17
  Risk for, 18

Loneliness, Risk for, 114

Memory, Impaired, 115

Mobility, Impaired
  Bed, 116
  Physical, 117
  Wheelchair, 119

Mucous membrane, Impaired oral, 127

Nausea, 120

Neglect, Unilateral, 121

Neurovascular dysfunction, Risk for peripheral, 136

Noncompliance, 122
Nutrition
    Imbalanced: Less than
      body requirements, 124
    Imbalanced: More than
      body requirements, 125
    Risk for imbalanced: More
      than body requirements,
      126
Oral mucous membrane,
    Impaired, 127
Organized infant behavior,
    Readiness for enhanced,
    107
Pain
    Acute, 129
    Chronic, 130
Parental role conflict, 46
Parent/infant/child attachment,
    Risk for impaired, 24
Parenting, Impaired, 131
    Risk for, 134
Perceived constipation, 51
Perioperative-positioning
    injury, Risk for, 111
Peripheral neurovascular dys
    function, Risk for, 136
Personal identity, Disturbed, 97
Physical mobility, Impaired, 117
Poisoning, Risk for, 137
Post-trauma syndrome, 138
    Risk for, 140
Powerlessness, 141
    Risk for, 142
Protection, Ineffective, 143
Rape-trauma syndrome, 144
    Compound reaction, 145
    Silent reaction, 146
Recovery, Delayed surgical, 181
Relocation stress syndrome, 147
    Risk for, 148

Retention, Urinary, 197
Role conflict, Parental, 46
Role performance, Ineffective,
    149
Role strain, Caregiver, 38
    Risk for, 41
Self-care deficit
    Bathing/hygiene, 151
    Dressing/grooming, 152
    Feeding, 153
    Toileting, 154
Self-esteem, Low, 156
    Chronic, 155
Situational, 156
    Risk for situational, 157
Self-mutilation, 158
    Risk for, 160
Sensory perception,
    Disturbed, 162
Sexual dysfunction, 163
Sexuality patterns, Ineffective,
    164
Skin integrity, Impaired, 165
    Risk for, 166
Sleep deprivation, 167
Sleep pattern, Disturbed, 169
Social interaction, Impaired, 172
Social isolation, 173
Sorrow, Chronic, 174
Spiritual distress, 175
    Risk for, 176
Spiritual well-being, Readiness
    for enhanced, 177
Suffocation, Risk for, 178
Suicide, Risk for, 179
Surgical recovery, Delayed, 181
Swallowing, Impaired, 182
Syndrome
    Disuse, Risk for, 67
    Environmental interpreta-
      tion, Impaired, 70

Syndrome *(continued)*
    Post-trauma, 138
    Risk for post-trauma, 140
    Rape-trauma, 144
    Rape-trauma, Compound
        reaction, 145
    Rape-trauma, Silent reaction,
        146
    Relocation stress, 147
Therapeutic regimen
    management
    Effective, 184
    Ineffective, 185
    Ineffective community, 186
    Ineffective family, 187
Thermoregulation, Ineffective,
    188
Thought processes, Disturbed,
    189
Tissue integrity, Impaired,
    190
Tissue perfusion, Ineffective,
    191
Toileting self-care deficit, 154
Transfer ability, Impaired, 193
Trauma, Risk for, 194
Unilateral neglect, 121

Urinary elimination, Impaired,
    196
Urinary incontinence
    Functional, 98
    Reflex, 99
    Risk for urge, 103
    Stress, 100
    Total, 101
    Urge, 102
Urinary retention, 197
Ventilation, Impaired sponta-
    neous, 198
Ventilatory weaning response,
    Dysfunctional, 199
Verbal communication,
    Impaired, 43
Violence, Risk for other-
    directed, 201
Violence, Risk for self-
    directed, 203
Walking, Impaired, 205
Wandering, 206
Weaning response,
    Dysfunctional ventila-
    tory, 199
Wheelchair mobility,
    Impaired, 119

Notes

Notes

Notes

Notes